The Future of Predictive Safety Evaluation

The Future of Predictive Safety Evaluation

In Two Volumes
Volume 1

Edited by
A.N. Worden
Cantab Group, Cambridge, England
D.V. Parke
Department of Biochemistry, University of Surrey, Guildford, England
J. Marks
Director of Medical Studies, Girton College, Cambridge, England

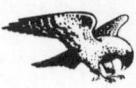 **MTP PRESS LIMITED**
a member of the KLUWER ACADEMIC PUBLISHERS GROUP
LANCASTER / BOSTON / THE HAGUE / DORDRECHT

Published in the UK and Europe by
MTP Press Limited
Falcon House
Lancaster, England

British Library Cataloguing in Publication Data

The Future of predictive safety evaluation.
    Vol. 1
1.   Toxicology---Technique   2.   Laboratory
animals
I. Worden, Alastair N.   II. Parke, Dennis, V.
III. Marks, John
613.9'00724   RA1199

ISBN-13: 978-94-010-8336-2   e-ISBN-13: 978-94-009-4139-7
DOI: 10.1007/978-94-009-4139-7

Published in the USA by
MTP Press
A division of Kluwer Academic Publishers
101 Philip Drive
Norwell, MA 02061, USA

Library of Congress Cataloging-in-Publication Data

The Future of predictive safety evaluation

Includes bibliographies and index
    1. Toxicity testing--Evaluation.   2. Health risk
    assessment--Evaluation.   I. Worden, Alastair N.
    II. Parke, Dennis V.   III. Marks, John, 1924-
    [DNLM: 1. Drugs--standards.   2. Drugs--toxicity.
    3. Environmental Monitoring--trends.   4. Environmental
    Pollutants--toxicity.   5. Environmental Pollution--
    prevention & control.   WA 670 F996]
    RA1199.F87   1986   363.1'79   86-10269
    ISBN-13: 978-94-010-8336-2

Contents

CONTENTS

PART 2 THE NEEDS (NON-PHARMACEUTICAL)

PART 3 PRECLINICAL: IN VITRO AND EX VIVO APPROACHES

Attribution

Several authors have asked us to state that the opinions expressed in their articles are personal and do not necessarily represent the official policy of their organizations. Rather than repeat this statement many times throughout the book, it should be regarded as applying to all the material submitted for publication.

List of
Contributors

Dr K.R. Butterworth
British Industrial Biological
Research Association
Carshalton
Surrey
England

Professor E.R. Carson
Director, Centre for Measurement
and Information in Medicine
The City University
London EC1
England

Dr D.M. Conning
British Industrial Biological
Research Association
Carshalton
Surrey
England

Professor M.A. Cooke
20 Kelmscott Road
Harborne
Birmingham
England

Dr B.J. Dean
32 The Poles
Upchurch
Sittingbourne
Kent
England

J.-M. Devos
Legal Counsellor
European Council of Chemical
Manufacturer's Federations
Avenue Louise 250, Bte 71
B-1050 Brussels
Belgium

Dr A.J. Dewar
Chemicals Planning
Shell Centre
London SE1
England

Dr E.L. Harris
Deputy Chief Medical Officer
Department of Health & Social
Security
London SE1
England

Dr W. Howe
Medical Department
ICI Organics Division
Manchester
England

Professor W.H.W. Inman
Director
Drug Surveillance Research Unit
University of Southampton
Southampton
England

Dr P. Knox
Department of Biochemistry
St George's Hospital Medical
School
London SW7
England

Dr J. Marks
Director of Medical Studies
Girton College
Cambridge
England

Dr K. Miller
Immunotoxicology Department
British Industrial Biological
Research Association
Carshalton
Surrey
England

S.Nicklin
Immunotoxicology Department
British Industrial Biological
Research Association
Carshalton
Surrey
England

Professor D.V. Parke
Department of Biochemistry
University of Surrey
Guildford
England

Dr J. Remfry
Universities Federation for
Animal Welfare
Potters Bar
Hertfordshire
England

Dr M.D. Stonard
Biomedical Sciences Section
Central Toxicology Laboratory
ICI
Alderley Park
Cheshire
England

Professor G. Teeling Smith
Office of Health Economics
London SW1
England

Dr. G.J. Turnbull
FBC Limited
Chesterford Park Research
Station
Saffron Walden
Essex
England

Dr N.J. Van Abbé
Research Department
Beecham Products
Weybridge
Surrey
England

Dr B.H. Woollen
Central Toxicology Laboratory
ICI
Alderley Park
Cheshire
England

Professor A.N. Worden
Cantab Group
Cambridge
England

Introduction

A. N. WORDEN, D. V. PARKE AND J. MARKS

THE BACKGROUND

There is nothing new about the fact that chemical substances derived either from natural products or by synthetic means can give rise to toxicity in animals and human beings, and that they must be subjected to controls. The earliest writings speak of such toxicity and, from the times of ancient Egypt and in the Old Testament, controls have existed[1].

In the Middle Ages Paracelsus (1493-1541) noted that "All things are poisons, for there is nothing without poisonous qualities. It is only the dose which makes a thing a poison", and hence he stressed the importance of dose relative to toxic reactions[2].

Most of the early controls concentrated on substances that were to be deliberately administered to the human subject in the form of medicines. Legislation for many centuries was mainly concerned with regulating the activities of apothecaries and physicians. The Royal College of Physicians, for example, was originally established to control the activities of physicians within London. Among the controls which it exerted was that over the use of medicinal substances. Such controls were, however, poor, based as they were on hearsay evidence of toxicity. For many centuries no means existed for the accurate determination of toxicity.

The first formal recognition of the subject of toxicology probably stems from the middle of the 19th century, when a course was given in Paris by Claude Bernard under the title "Lectures on the effects of toxic and medicinal subjects". This dealt with both noxious gases and natural substances[3].

The variety and availability of toxic substances has increased sharply since the close of the 19th century with intensive developments in the field of organic chemistry, and now there are many millions of substances which, taken in excess via the lungs, skin or mouth, can lead to morbidity or death.

Coupled with this increased number of potentially toxic sub-

1

stances that are available has come a dramatic increase in the ability to transmit information rapidly around the world, and with it a greater public awareness of toxicity. This stemmed largely from the dramatic and emotive story of thalidomide. Pressure groups of concerned people have also had the effect of heightening awareness. Hence the subject of toxicity appears now with great regularity in the medical and lay media, and the information is often presented in dramatic and exaggerated form. Yet epidemic poisoning is not confined to the present generation; for example in the Middle Ages ergotism was rife[4]. What is new is the greater awareness of the problems among both professionals and the lay public.

Toxicity may arise from a vast range of substances used in different ways and impinging on the body via various routes. Thus it can influence the body through the lungs (e.g. tobacco smoke), through the skin (e.g. radioactive substances, dioxan), through the alimentary canal in food (e.g. botulinus toxin, triorthocresyl phosphate in olive oil contaminated with petroleum oil), as pharmaceuticals (e.g. thalidomide) or as industrial chemicals (e.g. lead, benzene). In truth toxicity on a large scale, due to numerous chemical agents, has become a major worldwide social, ecological and economic problem[5]. Iatrogenic disease is now a major cause of hospitalization.

THE CURRENT SITUATION

National and international legal requirements

Legislation to control substances which may lead to toxicity has developed in a stepwise fashion over many years. The stage at which the different classes of compound (e.g. drugs, food, pesticides) have been covered by legislation has varied even within a single country. This depends on a variety of factors - some rational, some emotional. However the nature of the legislation and the rate at which it has been introduced varies even more widely from one country to another even within the industrially developed areas of the world.

In consequence national and international legal controls show marked variation. A single legal control covering the whole area of prevention of toxicity is virtually unknown in any country. In most there is a complicated set of laws often promulgated by different departments within the legislature.

Thus in the United Kingdom for example, drugs are currently controlled within regulations under the Medicines Act 1968, foods are still controlled under the Food and Drugs Act 1955, while chemical contaminants are largely controlled under the more recent Fertilizer and Feeding Stuffs Act 1976. Added to these there is a series of wider acts in which certain specific parts are concerned with toxicology. These include the Consumer Protection Act 1961, the Health and Safety at Work Act 1974 and the Radioactive Substances Act 1960. All of these cover a broader area of concern but have matters relevant to substance toxicity within them. A similar cluster of legislation is to be found in most industrialized countries. In contradistinction, many developing countries have only limited legal controls over substance toxicity.

International organizations, including the United Nations, the World Health Organization, and the European Economic Community, to name but three, have attempted to ensure that gross national differences in legislation are reduced and that a more logical arrangement of legal control shall exist. For example, various EEC directives have been issued from 1965 onwards in the area of medicines control.

While strenuous efforts are being made to exert a greater uniformity of sensible legal control, much still remains to be done in this area, and international control of potentially toxic substances is still a maze of legislation.

Even within the framework of existing legislation the extent of the implementation of the controls varies markedly from one country to another, depending upon social, philosophical, ethical and economic factors.

The current state of both national and international legislation and its application is far from ideal, and future broad international agreement, however difficult, is an essential factor in the further development of toxicology.

Present testing procedures and their relevance

Just as the legal controls differ from one country to another, so do the testing methods that are used, even for similar classes of substance, e.g. pesticides and drugs. When we consider inter-substance class situations, then the variation becomes even greater from one country to another. A majority of countries now insist on toxicological tests on new medicinal substances and on food. Controls related to pesticides and general chemicals may currently be less stringent in some countries. However the trend is towards international standardization of controls.

If one seeks test procedure similarities rather than differences, then most current substance tests are based upon acute, subacute and chronic toxicity studies in a variety of animal species. Until a few years ago acute toxicity studies formed a very large component of the overall testing procedure, but the relevance of the most widely used form, the LD_{50} or "lethal dose 50", is now in great doubt, and its use is being modified or dropped[6].

The selection of the animal species for such toxicity testing is often based upon such factors as economic cost, ease of husbandry and the avoidance of emotionally charged connotations, rather than on scientific logic. Small rodents are still the most common species that are used, yet the metabolism, nutrition and general behaviour of such animals is far removed from that of man that they are being used to predict, although not always more so than that of species closer to him phylogenetically. Until comparatively recently little effort has been made to match the test animals to the human subject on the basis of the metabolic and kinetic pattern of the substance to be tested, with the result that it is scarcely surprising that the predictive value of these tests has of-

3

ten been limited. For good reasons therefore the usefulness of much of the current routine toxicological testing has been sharply questioned[8].

Table 1 Suspensions and cancellations of licences for significant drugs in one or more European countries because of adverse effects (March 1982 to February 1984)

Benoxaprofen
Controlled release indomethacin (Osmosin, Indosmos)
Oxyphenbutazone
Phenylbutazone
Zomepirac
Zimelidine
Althesin*
Propanidid*
Methrasone

* Because of content of Cremophor EL.

The only relevant information in the last instance is experience in man. For pharmaceutical substances such human testing is an important component of premarketing activity. For other substances such premarketing testing is almost nonexistent or rare, even in the food area. Indeed legislation often makes it difficult or even impossible to undertake such studies, even on a volunteer basis.

Even with pharmaceutical products, however, recent experience has demonstrated that such premarketing testing does not necessarily provide a safety level that is acceptable to the community at large[9]. For example as Dukes has pointed out (Table 1) many drugs had their licences suspended or cancelled in one or more European countries in the 2 years from March 1982 because of adverse effects which were unsuspected in type or frequency during the trial stage.

In part it is inevitable that some substances which pass premarketing tests will fail when they are subjected to broad use. Premarketing testing rarely involves more than 10,000 patients yet, as Inman points out elsewhere in this book (Chapter 3), the use of 10,000 patients gives only a low confidence level of toxicity prediction. Thus for a study of 10,000 there is a 99% chance of recognizing toxicity at a level of 1 per 2000. This compares to the unacceptable toxicity level of, for example, zomepirac anaphylaxis, which is of the order of one death per two million patients (see also p. 51).

FACTORS INFLUENCING THE FUTURE

The sociopolitical environment

In most industrial countries the rate of population growth is declining and, at the same time, life expectancy is rising. This will alter the age structure of the population radically, and will particularly affect the proportion that the elderly form of the whole population. For example in the United Kingdom[10], whereas those over 65 formed 4.7% of the population at the turn of the century, they now (1985) form nearly 15%. Moreover the rise is due mainly to those that are very elderly and by 1990 those over 75 are likely to form almost 6.5% of the total population.

This means that, if we exclude the young and the old, only some 60% of the population will be wealth-creating, leading to difficulty in maintaining the gross national product (GNP). At the same time a greater proportion of the GNP will be devoted to health care. Thus for example in the USA health care cost represented 7.5% GNP in 1970, but by 1982 this figure had risen to 10.5%[11]. An increasingly ageing population will accentuate this problem, since old age is frequently associated with chronic poor health requiring extensive use of health-care services.

The increase in the proportion of the elderly will mean that greater attention will need to be paid to the toxic effects which are specific to that segment of the population. Recent experience has demonstrated that toxic reactions are more common in old age. This may be due to different pharmacokinetic patterns, e.g. indoprofen[12]. Hence there is bound to be a clash between the needs for toxicity determination and the means for accomplishing them. This problem will be increased by the specific need to develop pharmaceutical products which will deal with some of the problems of the elderly, and particularly those problems which lead to the greatest demand for the health-care services. Pharmaceutical therapy is inexpensive compared to hospital and social care costs. Thus unless there is a radical reappraisal of resource allocation the overall use of pharmaceutical products is likely to increase. Whether the present holistic approach will reverse this is a matter of conjecture.

A further socioeconomic factor which will affect future needs is the fact that global food demand will increase significantly - an increase by some 50-60% is predicted by the turn of the century. Most of this expansion will need to take place in developing countries, with yield enhancement an important aspect. This automatically implies that agrochemicals must become of greater importance, and that problems of testing for toxicity will be one important element in their development.

The recent high level of economic growth, with unprecedented utilization of resources coupled with developments in global communications, has led to an increased awareness of environmental issues. These in their turn have led to the emergence of environmental lobbies, and to an exceptional level of environmental concern in the population as a whole. As economic growth continues, with more countries aspiring to and achieving industrialization, the pressures on the environment will increase. Already in the developed world the marginal benefits of further growth are being increasingly compared by the "Green" lobbies with the adverse environmental consequences. Recent examples include the acid rain issue and the concern surrounding the disposal of hazardous chemical waste[6,13]. The risk of chemically induced cancer and teratogenicity tends to be of paramount importance in the public mind. Hence tests for mutagenicity, carcinogenicity and teratogenicity are assuming, or are likely to assume, a greater importance than might otherwise appear justified.

Allied to that relating to the environment, there is a growing pressure from within society for the reduction of animal experimentation. This pressure ranges from the increasingly militant activities of anti-vivisection groups, which are dedicated to the total abolition of animal experiments, to those of the more responsible animal welfare organizations to press for the so-called 3R's (Replacement of animal models, Reduction of the number of animals used, and the Refinement of toxicity tests[14]. Organizations such as FRAME permit an objective and scientific reappraisal of the aims and methodology of biomedical science and the development, validation and adoption of alternative techniques not involving live animal experimentation. There is a growing tendency for drug and chemical companies to develop guidelines emphasizing humane treatment and minimum use of animals, and many are now dedicated to, and have published, developments on so-called alternative test procedures.

The industrial environment

The current world recession, coupled with high levels of inflation and high energy costs, have led to severe cutbacks in the chemical industry, particularly the petrochemical industry in which there was gross over-capacity. At the same time there is increased competition from low-cost production in newly industrialized countries. In the future it is likely that more and more of the bulk chemicals and chemical intermediates will come from these newer producing centres. The older industrialized communities will then need to rely more upon further chemical developments and research. This will inevitably mean that the development costs will fall more avily on the industrialized countries, and these costs will include those for toxicological testing. Toxicological testing and postmarketing surveillance for toxic reactions are likely to be minimal for the older chemicals. If these older chemicals are produced to a high state of purity, such that the previous data are appropriate, then there will be relatively few inherent risks (medical, social, economic) in the situation, providing international patent law is observed. This would allow adequate return on development costs for those in the older industrialized countries and encourage the relevant research which is necessary.

INTRODUCTION

Experience over the past few years has demonstrated that, although some of the newer manufacturing communities achieve a high state of purity in their products, this is not universally the case. Hence there may be concern in the future about the validity of existing toxicological data and a need for more careful community screening for toxic effects of commonly used bulk chemicals. This is of particular concern in relation to fertilizers.

Coupled with this change there will be a growing emphasis in the older industrialized countries on the development, investigation and production of a large range of relatively small-volume novel chemicals, some of which will pose new problems of toxicological assessment[15,16].

The scientific and technological environment

Adherents of the controversial long-wave theory first proposed by Kondratiev in 1935 have claimed that basic innovations common to all industry occur in clusters at intervals of roughly 50 years. Long-wave theorists such as Mensch believe that since the late 1940s the frequency of major innovations has declined, but that a new wave of innovation is likely to occur in the 1990s[17]. Most observers would concur with the view that the pace of major product innovation in the chemical and pharmaceutical industries has declined sharply in recent decades. Whether this is due to the macroeconomic forces of the long-wave theorists or to the escalating costs of research development is a matter of dispute[15].

Even if one does not accept the long-wave hypothesis, the proposition that a new wave of chemical innovation could occur at the end of this century is a tenable one[19,20]. Basic research techniques such as computer modelling, receptor structure activity and the development of powerful new instrumental techniques and analytical tools based upon the rapidity of action of microelectronic control mechanisms are becoming a powerful stimulus to greater ease of research. Of particular significance have been radical advances in catalysis[21] and the emergence of computational quantum chemistry[22]. The inability to solve the immensely complicated equation has been an enormous stumbling block in quantum chemistry for nearly half a century. The advent of powerful high-speed computers has made a practical possibility of chemical experimentation via computer calculations rather than direct laboratory work. This is beginning to have a marked influence in such fields as drug and agrochemical development.

The other development which may have an equally large influence in the closing years of the present century is the field of biotechnology. The key biotechnological inventions of the last 15 years (recombinant DNA, monoclonal antibodies and immobilized enzyme technology) will confer a considerable potential ability to the whole chemical industry to harness biological processes towards the generation of new products and new processes[23].

Risk perception

One current recent aspect which will influence the future is that of the perception of risk and attempts at its quantification. People respond to the hazards which they perceive and their appreciation of their probability. This perception is in part rational, dependent on past experience (whether or not this is valid for future prediction) and in part dependent on subjective judgement[24]. Despite an appearance of objectivity all forms of risk assessment include a subjective component. As might be expected the perceived level of risk varies with the expertise of the assessing group[24]. The wider the general knowledge about the factors involved in the risk the greater has been the agreement between lay and expert groups.

The acceptance of risk when it has been defined shows marked variation[25]. Harvey gives as an example the fact that Californians will continue to live happily on the San Andreas fault, but protest vehemently against a lesser nuclear venture risk. Members of the public also apply qualitative judgements to particular risks, e.g. radioactivity and carcinogenicity, and also expect a higher standard for occupational risks that are not seen as voluntary. On the other hand some man-made risks (e.g. road deaths) are accepted at a much greater level.

Logically it would be anticipated that risk acceptance would bear a relationship to the perception of the benefit to be equated with it, but this does not seem to apply in practice[24]. For example the limit of risk acceptability of vaccination would appear to be about 10^{-6} under non-epidemic circumstances, irrespective of the variable risks inherent in different infections. The acceptable risk for medications appears to be of the same order.

Since the principle of toxicology is that it should assess risk before human exposure starts, it follows that factors which affect the assessment and acceptance of risk <u>in the minds of the lay public</u> are paramount in defining the extent and scope of toxicological study. It is the lay public, and particularly pressure groups in the lay public, who exert the major influence over the legislative activities of a government on safety.

From this it follows that developments in risk assessment will be of major future significance and it behoves industrialists and those concerned with the economic aspects of toxicological testing to attempt to educate the public towards a more rational and less emotional appraisal of risk acceptance.

PROBLEMS OF THE FUTURE TO BE SOLVED

This book is concerned with predictions on how problems in toxicological testing, which it is anticipated will occur during the rest of this century, may be approached or solved. Broadly the anticipated problems may be divided into three areas.

INTRODUCTION

Poor prediction from toxicological testing

Reference has already been made to the fact that many of the current toxicological tests have relatively poor prediction value. In part this results from the fact that even a low incidence of substance toxicity is usually unacceptable. In part it stems from difficulties over validating current methods. The greatest chance of validation lies in the field of drugs. The human subject is exposed to new drugs under controlled conditions during clinical testing. Then subsequently, at the marketing stage, there is reasonable information on the extent of the exposure. Validation for substances that are not intended for human ingestion is much more difficult to achieve.

Animal toxicological testing remains difficult to validate among pharmaceuticals, and is even more difficult in other areas: its probable future role and its place within the context of overall appraisal are discussed in the relevant chapters.

The development of new chemical entities

Current methods of toxicological testing are based on a certain amount of validation within the field of existing chemical usage and exposure, whether this be deliberate or by accident.

The developments in chemistry, and particularly in biotechnology, are likely to result in an entirely new range of substances before the end of the century. Unfortunately we have no means of knowing whether the existing toxicological methods will be adequate to determine unusual toxic effects which may occur from these new chemical classes.

We may take the analogy of thalidomide which was subjected to the then currently validated toxicological tests before being introduced to the market and, within these tests, showed itself to be a very safe compound. It was only after human teratogenic effects had emerged that it was appreciated that the current tests as applied to drugs were inadequate to demonstrate this effect. Indeed it was only when certain species of animal, and a new regime, were used that the experimental determination of the teratogenic effect of thalidomide became possible.

We must recognize that an effect like that exerted by thalidomide, be it specific organ toxicity, teratogenicity or carcinogenicity, may occur with other compounds in the future despite current methods of testing. The greater the difference between the new chemical class and those that have been validated, the greater the potential risk. This implies that, while toxicological methods should involve the use of validated techniques, both currently available and developed in the future, the only final protection against tragedies of the type demonstrated by thalidomide is the epidemiological examination of changes in mortality and morbidity. Such studies are, however, difficult for, as in the case of the carcinogenic effect of smoking, morbidity may only occur after prolonged exposure of possibly one or two decades after such exposure. Hence one vital aspect of development in toxicology is a first-class epidemiological monitoring system. With the new computer-based data acquisition this should be feasible.

Economic aspects of toxicology

Current testing procedures are expensive, both in terms of time and money. As industrially developing nations move further into chemical manufacture, greater emphasis will be placed in the older industrialized countries on research developments and the recoupment of the costs of research within the patent life.

In most countries the patent life is measured from the date of first registration. Extension of the patent life, if it can be accomplished, only provides a relatively short additional period (usually of the order of 4 years). At the present time the longest period for full animal and human toxicological and safety study lies in the pharmaceutical field. This testing programme currently takes at least 10 years when any prolonged human exposure is anticipated. This effectively reduces the period of marketing within the original patent life to under half.

With increased concern about the toxic effects of other chemicals (e.g. fertilizers, food additives, general chemicals) it is likely that more extensive toxicology will be demanded. This will increase research and development costs in these areas too and, by encroaching on the patent life, will diminish the potential return on research costs.

By changing toxicological methods, and by better programming, it may be possible to achieve some reduction in the length of time required for toxicological testing, but unfortunately the reduction is not likely to be substantial. In the circumstances it would appear that the best possibility for appropriate financial return on research expenditure will come from a modification of patent law, perhaps by the provision of a more limited but defined number of years **after** development is complete.

STRUCTURE OF THIS BOOK

This book has been structured to attempt, through the efforts of the many contributors, to show what each of them feels could or should be done to predict safety in the use of, or from exposure to, substances that are ingested by man or with which he otherwise may come into contact. A varying amount of space has inevitably been devoted to past and present shortcomings of testing and assessment procedures, but the emphasis is upon the future. The task of prediction is extremely complex and is complicated by the fact that the degree of intrinsic toxicity in a conventional sense is not inversely related to safety in use. It will be evident, as already indicated, that the general or systemic toxicity of thalidomide is of a low order. Yet it was the untoward effects of this compound in use that did more to excite professional, political and lay concern, and to promote regulatory and quasi-regulatory activity, than any other factor to date.

Division of the work into several Parts within two Volumes is of necessity somewhat arbitrary, but the groupings permit of an appraisal of categories of compounds and of a disciplinary approach to their study respectively. Interspersed is a Part (in Volume 2) devoted to the molecular aspects of toxicity prediction. In some respects this approach may prove to be the key to what can be attempted in future years. It should lead to far better understanding of differences between species, including man, and between individuals within a species. It could relate, much more convincingly than is currently possible, in vitro with in vivo models. Combined with non-invasive techniques and other approaches already mentioned, it could greatly enhance the value of tests on man himself - and on other animal models should these still prove to be necessary. That they probably will be, albeit in modified and reduced form, is the opinion of the authors of the relevant chapters - at least for some decades to come.

REDUCING RISK BY LIMITING EXPOSURE

This book is primarily concerned with the methods which may be adopted over the next decade for the assessment of risk **before** human exposure occurs. It also stresses that, however good these methods may be, the risk assessment must continue after commercial availability by appropriate epidemiological studies. This information will modify the assessment which has been made. With appropriate validation it may be hoped that the level of accuracy of risk assessment will steadily increase.

However, actual damage only occurs after exposure has occurred. Hence it is important to define the advised level of exposure to any chemical. This should be related to the balance of social benefit and the estimated risk. Hence the eventual need is for risk-benefit analysis rather than just risk assessment. This applies irrespective of whether we are considering an industrial chemical or a drug with a highly specific therapeutic activity.

Ultimately it should be this risk-benefit factor which should determine both the level of legislative control and the educational effort that is needed.

REFERENCES

1. Penn, RG (1979). The state control of medicines: the first 3000 years. J Clin Pharmacol, 8, 293-305
2. Cited in Sigerist, HE (1958). The Great Doctors. (New York: Doubleday)
3. Bernard, C (1857). Lecons sur les Effets des Substances Toxiques et Medicamenteuses. (Paris: J-B Bailliere et Fils)
4. Barger, G (1931). Ergot and Ergotism. (London: Gurney & Jackson)
5. Carson, R (1962). Silent Spring. (Boston: Houghton Mifflin)
6. Anon (1984). Animals in testing; how the CPI is handling a hot issue. Chemical Week, 5 December, pp. 36-40
7. Brimblecombe, RW and Dayan, AD (1985). Preclinical toxicity testing. Pharmaceutical Medicine, 36. (London: Edward Arnold)

8. Zbinden, G (1966). Animal toxicity studies: a critical evaluation. Appl Ther, 8, 128

9. Dukes, G (1985). The Effects of Drug Regulation. (Lancaster: MTP Press)

10. Data from Department of Health and Social Services Statistical Publications. London: HMSO

11. Haunalter, G (1983). Health Issues and Trends in the 1980s. Stanford Research International Report No. 689

12. Kurowski, M (1985). Pharmocokinetics of indoprofen in elderly patients following repeated oral administration. Int J Clin Pharmacol Res, 5, 255-63

13. Jones, JL (1980). Disposal of Hazardous Waste - a Major Environmental Issue for the 1980s. Stamford Research Report No. 637

14. Rowan, AN (1983). Alternatives: Interaction between science and animal welfare. In Goldberg, AM (ed) Product Safety Evaluation. pp. 113-33. (New York: MA Liebert)

15. Malpas, R (1982). A "geochemical" view of the year 2000. In Sharp, DH and West, TF (eds). The Chemical Industry. pp. 99-117. (London: Ellis Horwood)

16. Harvey-Jones, JH (1983). New directions for the chemical industry. Chemistry & Industry, 923-6.

17. Mensch, GO (1979). Statement in Technology: Innovations Overcome Depression. (Cambridge, Mass.: Ballinger/Harper & Row)

18. Graham, AK and Senge, PM (1980). A long wave hypothesis of innovation. Technol Forecasting Soc Change, 17, 283-311

19. Robertson, NC (Chairman of Expert Panel) (1982). A new wave - is a new golden age of chemical innovation on the way? Chem Strategies, 1, 16-28

20. Wells, N (1983). Pharmaceutical Innovation: Recent Trends, Future Prospects. (London: Office of Health Economics)

21. Maugh, TH (1983). Catalysis: no longer a black art. Science, 219, 474-7

22. Wilson, S (1982). Chemistry by computer. New Scientist, 576-9

23. Bull, AT, Holt G and Lilly, MD (1982). Biotechnology - International Trends and Perspectives. (Paris: OECD)

24. Slovic, P, Fischhoff, B and Lichtenstein, S (1981). Perceived risk: psychological factors and social implications. Proc R Soc Lond, A376, 17-34

25. Harvey, PG (1981). An industralist's attitude to risk. Proc R Soc Lond, A376, 193-7

PART 1
General Considerations

1
Toxicology: Regulatory Authority Requirements

E. L. HARRIS

Some 6 million chemical substances have so far been identified, 80% of them in the past 40 years. Between 50,000 and 70,000 of these 6 million substances are in use at the present time. In addition, about 10,000 entities are discovered each month[1]. Society expects - or rather demands - that chemicals in use, or present in the environment, are evaluated for safety. It is not possible to cover in a short chapter all the legislative and other controls that are concerned with the safety of chemicals for which governments have a responsibility. I will concentrate on current regulations in the United Kingdom and attempt to predict possible future toxicological requirements.

The principal controls have been introduced in a series of measures over many years. The main ones are:

1. The Food and Drugs Act 1955 [2]
This seeks to ensure that the consumer can buy safe, wholesome food and is not misled about its character or quality. Regulations made under the powers conferred by this Act have been used to establish standards in slaughterhouses, docks, markets, mobile shops, stalls, delivery vehicles and food premises. There are also regulations controlling:

(a) the composition of certain foodstuffs;
(b) the additives and processing aids that may be present;
(c) the amounts of certain components (e.g. lead) present in food;
(d) the labelling and advertizing of foods to be sold.

The contents of this chapter represent the author's views alone and in no way commit the Department of Health and Social Security

THE FUTURE OF PREDICTIVE SAFETY EVALUATION

2. The Medicines Act 1968 [3]

This provides for a comprehensive licensing system for the marketing, manufacture, importation and clinical testing of medicinal products for both human and veterinary use. Licences are issued by a Licensing Authority which consists of the Health and Agriculture Ministers of the UK. The Licensing Authority is advised by independent expert committees set up under powers in the Act which take into account the safety, quality and efficacy of medicinal products. These committees are known as Section 4 Committees. They are statutory and comprise the Committee on Safety of Medicines, the Committee on the Review of Medicines, the Committee on Dental and Surgical Materials, the Veterinary Products Committee and the British Pharmacopoeia Commission.

The Medicines Act also established the Medicines Commission, which is a statutory body with members from the medical, veterinary and pharmacy professions, as well as chemists and members from the pharmaceutical industry. It gives advice to Ministers on general matters relating to the implementation of the Act, and on medicines in general. It also acts as an appellate body when applicants for clinical trial certificates or product licences make representations against an adverse recommendation by one of the Section 4 Committees.

The Licensing Authority has a continuing role in monitoring the safety of drugs that are being clinically evaluated, as well as all products that have been marketed. It is also responsible for controlling the promotion and advertizing of products, and for setting standards of good manufacturing practice. The British Pharmacopoeia Commission is responsible for setting standards for human and veterinary medicines and publishes the "British armacopoeia" and the "British Pharmacopoeia (Veterinary)".

Additional controls in the medicines field originated from European Community Directives. Directives 65/65, 75/318, and 75/319 were formulated with the aim of harmonizing the control of medicines in member states. Directive 75/318, known as the "standards and protocol" directives, sets out the type of information required to license a new medicinal product and covers minimal standards for chemistry, pharmacy, pharmacology, toxicology and clinical trials. At present it does not cover biological products such as vaccines. Directive 75/319 establishes a Committee for Proprietary Medicinal Products with each member state being represented by an official concerned with licensing. The Committee gives advice on products licensed in one country where applications have been made to other countries, and also advises on particular products which are referred to it. The Pharmaceutical Committee is responsible for advising on general matters concerning medicines, including the revision of existing directives.

16

3. Fertiliser and Feeding Stuffs Act 1976 [4]

As amended, this Act covers inter alia the presence of chemical contaminants in compounded animal feeding stuffs as well as vitamin and mineral supplementation.

A variety of other controls, such as the Radioactive Substance Act 1964[5] the Health and Safety at Work Act 1974[6] and its regulations, the Consumer Protection Act 1961[7], and EC directives are all designed to protect the public. In addition, a number of officially agreed voluntary schemes relate to chemicals in the environment. The Pesticide Safety Protection Scheme was introduced to protect the user of a pesticide, but it also takes into account any environmental effects on wildlife and on the human food chain.

Apart from dealing with medicinal products the Department of Health and Social Security has a general responsibility within Government for toxicological advice on:

(a) substances for use in food, including food additives, processing aids and food constituents derived from novel sources;

(b) food contaminants, naturally occurring toxins in food and food contaminants, including substances which may originate from packaging materials and residues of pesticides and veterinary products;

(c) cosmetics and toiletries;

(d) household products and other consumer products, including some industrial chemicals;

(e) environmental pollutants;

(f) chemicals used in the formulation of medicines.

The Department is advised by a number of expert committes made up of independent outside specialists. The main committees are:

1. Committee on Toxicity of Chemicals in Food, Consumer Products and the Environment[8].

2. Committee on Carcinogenicity[9].

3. Committee on Mutagenicity[10].

4. Advisory Committee on Irradiated and Novel Foods.

5. Committee on Contamination of Air, Soil and Water.

Advice is requested from other government departments, mainly the Ministry of Agriculture, Fisheries and Food which is advised on the Food and Drug Act by the Food Advisory Committee. There is a further expert committee on pesticides which advises on the operation of the voluntary Pesticides Safety Precautions Scheme. This is a non-statutory but formally negotiated scheme under which every formulation destined to be marketed in the UK is first

THE FUTURE OF PREDICTIVE SAFETY EVALUATION

scrutinized for the safety to the user, potential residues in food and effects on wildlife.

Members of these advisory committees are independent experts from scientific disciplines such as medicine, veterinary practice, pharmacy, chemistry and microbiology. They come from universities, private practice and industry. Consumer interests are also represented. These experts are selected for their experience in scrutinizing data and assessing human health risk. The committees have produced flexible guidelines with the object of assisting industry in describing the nature of the data to be submitted and the form in which the data are required. It is recognized that absolute safety can never be proved by any system of tests. The assessment of any hazard to man depends upon the interpretation of animal and other laboratory studies in the context of human exposure. The extent and nature of the studies necessary to support the safety-in-use of a chemical depends on many factors, and therefore the tests required for a particular substance will vary from those needed for a chemical in another category. The object of the guidance is to enable an informed assessment to be made of any risks to man, whilst at the same time limiting the amount of animal experimentation needed.

As new technologies are developed which result in new or novel products further guidance is needed. It may be enough to update existing guidance but in some cases new advice must be offered. The "Memorandum on the Testing of Novel Foods"[11] issued by the UK Health Departments and MAFF, containing the advice of the Expert Advisory Committee on Irradiated and Novel Foods is a good example of this situation. The memorandum, which has been produced for the guidance of companies interested and in developing or marketing novel foods (including foods produced by novel processes), points out that the traditional method of assessing the safety of food additive, i.e. allowing a 100-fold margin between the maximum amount of an additive likely to be consumed in the human diet and the maximum amount which has no toxic effect when fed to animals, clearly cannot be applied to a novel food which would constitute more than 1% of the human diet. In any case there are practical limits to the amounts of certain foods which can be added to animal diets without adversely affecting the animals' nutritional status and health. The guidance also states that once a novel food has been adequately tested in appropriate animal and in vitro systems it should always undergo tolerance testing, which includes monitoring for possible allergenicity in small groups of normal human volunteers under controlled conditions and under medical supervision. The emphasis of the guidelines is on flexibility rather than on laying down specific requirements for the studies with which it deals.

The approach to the control of chemicals in food has been clearly described by Bunyon, Coomes and Elton[12]. They dealt with the philosophy of risk to health and risk management techniques. The government's role in the case of food is to ensure that it is safe. Risk management for the government involves identifying and estimating the risks associated with the consumption of food, putting them in context with the other risks to life and reducing them to a practicable minimum for the population at large by legislation or other means, as appropriate.

The advisory committee and government officials are involved with risk assessment decisions, and in the case of foods, additives and contaminants, controls must be suited to the needs of consumers and should not overburden the chemical or food industry with undue costs in order to provide data which allow the decisions about risk to be taken. It would be fair to say that since the last war the advice of the independent expert committees on regulatory controls on food and food additives, in respect of both consumer and industry, has served the country well.

One of the important safeguards introduced in the past two decades has been the conduct of regular reviews and re-appraisals of regulations carried out at the request of Ministers. These are drawn up by the expert committees and involve consultation with manufacturers, consumers and the enforcement authorities. The reports are published and are available for scrutiny even after the formal consultation has taken place before publication.

In the case of medicinal products the advisory committee structure has already been described. The Licensing Authority is advised by medical, veterinary and pharmaceutical assessors. Detailed guidance on requirements for applications either for the clinical trial or field trials of products is provided[13]. The guidance is aimed to help applicant companies provide the necessary data in a clear format. The emphasis overall is that each new product requires data which are determined by the product's intended use. There is a continuing process of review and reassessment of requirements and guidance. In some instances these follow the deliberations of a special group set up by the Committee on Safety of Medicines, such as Professor Grahame Smith's Working Party on Toxicity Requirements for Medicinal Products. A regular dialogue also takes place with individual companies making application, as well as with the appropriate trade associations. The Medicines Commission oversees the work of the Section IV Committees. Contact with regulators worldwide takes place at governmental level, firstly within the European Community through the Pharmaceutical Committee and the Committee on Proprietary Medicinal Products. Early after its formation the latter set up a working party on requirements for toxicological testing. This has resulted in EC guidelines which have gone a long way towards harmonizing requirements within the Community.

The United Kingdom regulators hold annual meetings with senior officials of the American Food and Drug Administration and the Canadian Health and Welfare Department. These meetings, which started off on an informal basis, are now known as the Tripartite Meetings and are extremely useful for exchanging views on requirements for toxicological evaluation and methods of risk-benefit assessment on both sides of the Atlantic. There is great mutual benefit in such an arrangement and it can result in collaborative efforts involving other countries. A good example of this was action which took place as a result of long-term rat studies carried out in Japan on the permitted anti-oxidant, butylated hydroxyanisole (BHA)[14]. Proposed Japanese regulatory action against this food additive could have had a significant effect in the Common Market and North America, but because of the close collaboration which produced a detailed review of all the safety evidence on this compound, the decision was reached to allow BHA to be used in food until further defined work has been carried out.

Apart from the Common Market countries, regular contact is maintained with regulatory authorities in the Nordic countries and other European countries outside the EC. The World Health Organization also has a role to play, mainly in fostering exchanges between experts and by promoting the publication of expert advice. The Organization also sponsors the meetings, now on a biennial basis, of the International Conference of Drug Regulatory Authorities.

PREDICTIONS OF FUTURE TRENDS IN REGULATORY CONTROL

Demographic changes that will occur in the population by regulatory controls need to be examined. Goldberg[15] pointed out that toxicological studies have until now used normal healthy animals as models for the totality of the human population. Little attention has been paid hitherto to the problems posed for children, the disabled and the elderly. All over the world the proportion of the elderly and disabled in the population is growing significantly. In Britain the proportion over the age of 65 years will be 32%, and 1.9% will be over 85 years[16] when we reach the turn of the century. As more diseases are conquered life expectancy will increase for those who may have different sensitivity to chemicals to which the exposure of the population as a whole is considered safe.

With better education and improvements in mass communication more members of the public will expect to be better protected by regulatory controls. Demands are likely to intensify over the next 20 years. Whenever patients are harmed by drugs and regulatory action is taken, either by restricting their use or withdrawing them from the market, vociferous demands are made for the introduction of more controls. Dukes[17] has observed that the debate on drug regulation has been conducted largely at the political and industrial level with more recent participation from the consumer movement. The discussions were mainly on matters of principle with emotional arguments playing a major role.

Cause and effect relationships have remained unproved, if only because many of the essential data on risks and effective means of avoiding them have not been available. Policymakers have not therefore been able to form an objective view of the regulations needed by society, and their decisions may have been determined largely by the various pressures brought to bear on them. Expectations of society for safety protection apply equally as much to flying or transport by rail or road. In this case the public is able to perceive the risk and can exert appropriate pressures on policymakers to introduce regulatory controls.

In looking at future regulatory requirements in the field of toxicology, I agree with the views of Goldberg[15], who stated "I find myself a strange bedfellow among the Futurists. For the most part they are doomsayers. . . . As far as toxicology can influence the environmental and human condition I find much cause for optimism; in fact I feel that there has never been a time of such ferment and so much promise." Cromie[18] drew attention to the fact that when new procedures were introduced older tests were not abandoned, thus the burden on industry increased with each new discovery. He calculated the effect the regulatory controls would have in future, and predicted that for one of the largest multinational pharmaceutical companies innovatory activities would cease before the year 2000. I am optimistic about the future and believe that commonsense attitudes will prevail. We have already seen that there is a far more questioning approach to standard tests. Requirements for those that are found to be wanting, such as the LD-50, are being modified or dropped altogether[19].

There is a general consensus that there does not at present appear to be any possibility of replacing long-term whole animal studies. Attitudes about these investigations are changing, and the requirement that they be extended for longer than 6 months is gradually being dropped except in the case of carcinogenicity studies. There is increased interest in the mechanism by which toxic effects are produced. This means that the days of the rigid checklist approach to safety testing are numbered.

It is possible to make predictions about what Regulatory Authorities will require in future for animal toxicity studies on the basis of experience over the past 20 years, and to take into account the inherent conservative nature of the regulators. Whilst little change has occurred in requirements for standard preclinical tests such as acute, subacute and chronic studies over the past 20 years, variations have been introduced mainly based on the nature of the chemical to be evaluated.

Twenty years ago carcinogenicity studies were not a regular

THE FUTURE OF PREDICTIVE SAFETY EVALUATION

requirement before human exposure was permitted. Mutagenicity testing had not yet appeared. Although tests relating to mutagenicity are now a standard component of safety testing the interpretation of their significance is still subject to uncertainty and doubt.

There is a healthy tendency for the value of all these tests in predicting safety in man to be examined critically, but relevant data are not easily obtained and significant departures from these tests are unlikely in the next 20 years.

In the case of pharmaceutical products the main change will occur by attempts to harmonize requirements for drug regulation. In Europe this will develop at two levels: the first within the Common Market and the second by the World Health Organization. The aim of the Common Market is to allow the free movement of products between member states by removal of barriers to free trade. Since the establishment of the Committee for Proprietary Medicinal Products in 1975 there have been two proposals to remove obstacles to free trade[19]. The first is a scheme for the mutual recognition of decisions taken by national regulatory authorities. Progress along these lines will now be slow, mainly because of differences in philosophy on diseases and the therapeutic approach to them. The example that is regularly quoted is the French concept of hepatic dysfunction and the use of liver tonics for its treatment, which receive little or no recognition in the United Kingdom and across the Atlantic. The second proposal is the establishment of a Community Drug Regulatory Authority. Whilst this has attractions in that unnecessary duplication of work in each member state would be reduced, there is a real underlying fear that a vast and ineffective bureaucratic machine would result which would delay the introduction of new pharmaceuticals. There is further evidence to support this view based on the experience of the Benelux countries. In 1972 Belgium, Holland and Luxembourg established a Registration Authority to provide a single system for drug control in the three countries. It was found that assessments of applications received by the new Authority were carried out far slower than in each member state, and this, compounded by the adoption of a higher standard for nearly all requirements, resulted in a high incidence of refusals. Pharmaceutical companies, recognizing that it was easier to obtain clearance through a member state, abandoned attempts to obtain simultaneous registration through the new Authority. Some improvements to the system were attempted but had little effect, and in 1982 the scheme was abandoned. Extrapolation from this experience does not suggest that a single regulatory authority for the Common Market could function satisfactorily unless attitudes change significantly. Over the next 20 years this is unlikely. We ought to be moving to the situation where the onus is clearly on the individual country to show why it needs to stand out against the views of the majority. In this

22

sense I expect to see a movement towards harmonization of decisions, although over a relatively long timescale.

The one area where I would confidently predict an early change in Common Market requirements is in the field of biological products. At the moment these are not covered by existing directives. It is illogical that this is so, and in my view it is only a matter of time before they are brought under regulatory control by a new directive. This will also become more important as a result of the introduction of products based on high-technology advances mainly in the field of biotechnology. A further extension of EC requirements is likely to include compliance with the principles of good laboratory practice in all fields where there are toxicological requirements. This is a logical extension of the practice adopted by most member states at the present time.

The World Health Organization, since its foundation in 1948, has had an interest in pharmaceutical products. In recent years there has been growing pressure within the Organization to set up what can be regarded as an International Regulatory Authority. This has found little favour with the membership. However, in recent years the European Region has accepted the task of examining this possibility in greater detail. In 1981 a draft proposal for international collaboration was submitted by the Secretariat to the Annual Regional Assembly. The proposal was based on a scheme in which a pharmaceutical company would apply to the Drug Evaluation Unit in Copenhagen for a Scientific Evaluation Document (SED). The basis of the scheme was the concept that the drug evaluation unit act as a drug regulatory authority. The scheme was vigorously opposed at the Annual Assembly and various toned-down proposals were put forward based on WHO acting as a centre for distribution of information on drugs. The main reason why the SED scheme was not favoured was because the Organization could not guarantee confidentiality of data. Other concerns were that an extensive bureaucracy would evolve (q.v. the reaction to the proposal for the establishment of an EC Regulatory Authority), that diverse philosophical approaches to drug regulation would cause unnecessary delays, and that rising standards of requirements would result in more frequent rejections of applications.

Although for the moment the idea of either a European or world regulatory authority has been shelved there are some within the Organization and in member states who will continue to promote its development. They feel that whilst developed countries can be satisfied with their own regulatory activities, the main beneficiaries of a WHO scheme would be the developing countries which do not have the financial or manpower resources to establish their own national controls. But this assumes that all countries have the same needs for controls on medicines, whereas this would depend not only on pattern of disease in the country but on the state of development of its health services. The WHO/FAO Joint Expert

THE FUTURE OF PREDICTIVE SAFETY EVALUATION

Committee on Food Additives and Contaminants is not a regulatory body but provides advice on acceptable daily intakes of chemicals in foods. This is of great benefit to countries who do not have the resources to make their own assessments of safety.

Pressure from the increasingly active animal protection groups, and the recognition that animal studies - although valuable in revealing many safety problems - have limitations for assessing safety for man suggests that regulatory authorities will in future require more data on humans before giving authorization for marketing. This will result in two developments. There will be a gradual rise in the requirements for volunteer (normal subjects) studies over longer periods of time. It is likely that the demands for these additional studies will not initially be incorporated into legislative requirements, but will be necessary because of the need to satisfy authorities on safety. Similarly more clinical trials involving larger numbers of patients over longer periods of time will gradually become the norm.

This trend towards an increase in the number of clinical studies required before a product is marketed becomes evident when one compares Advisory Committee requirements 20 years ago with those of the present day. The withdrawal of practalol ("Eraldin") tablets in 1976 as a result of the development of an oculomucocutaneous syndrome in patients taking the drug and, more recently, of some non-steroid anti-inflammatory agents, for example benoxaprofen ("Opren") have had, and will increasingly have, the effect of emphasizing the need for more premarketing clinical studies.

In the case of newer novel foods I have already mentioned that the Advisory Committee has given clear-cut guidance on requirements for studies in humans[11]. This guidance deals with preliminary single-dose studies, longer-term investigations of about 4 weeks' duration and prolonged follow-up procedures.

It is also stated that if a novel food is intended to be eaten by a certain group of people (for example diabetics) at least one study should be conducted on people from that group. When a novel food's safety has been demonstrated by these rather limited studies large-scale acceptability and marketing trials should be undertaken, paying particular attention to vulnerable groups such as pregnant women, children, the elderly and any other group at risk, such as persons with an inborn error of metabolism.

POSTMARKETING SURVEILLANCE

There is little doubt that demands will continue to be made for more effective postmarketing surveillance for all new products. I am not sanguine that much improvement in existing schemes will occur in the next two decades. The main reason for this is that resources will continue to be restricted and, more importantly, the methodology of surveillance still has many deficiencies.

It is likely that regulatory authorities will require greater effort by marketing companies for postmarketing surveillance of their products. These will inevitably impose financial and manpower burdens on industry, and past experience, certainly in the field of pharmaceutical products, suggests that some will be of limited value but others would help to clarify uncertainties about safety. A good example is the study on cimetidine[21], in which 9928 patients taking the drug and 9311 controls were followed up to 1 year. The study successfully detected and quantified some already known adverse effects of cimetidine and did not detect any new effects. The authors concluded that this method of postmarketing surveillance is feasible and useful, but that data interpretation is complicated.

CONCLUSION

I am optimistic that regulatory authorities will avoid unnecessary restrictions on industry, and that the need for flexibility in setting testing requirements will continue while still attaching primary importance to protecting the health of the consumer. I believe that there will be important advances in our ability to detect adverse reactions, especially through developments in premarketing clinical studies. However, this will not mean that we shall pass out of the time when quite unexpected adverse reactions occur. The wider use of products of all kinds which are technically sophisticated, and which bring many benefits, almost inevitably means that there will also be, perhaps only for limited groups who are particularly vulnerable, adverse effects which were not, and probably could not have been, foreseen. The increasing challenge for the future will be in taking decisions about the relationship between risk and benefit and the action which it is appropriate for the community to take in individual instances.

REFERENCES

1.   Lonngren, R (1984). Rules and Regulations World Health, Aug./Sept., p.28
2.   Medicines Act 1968 (CH 67). (London: HMSO)
3.   Food and Drugs Act 1955 (4 Eliz. 2 C 16). (London: HMSO)
4.   Fertilizer and Feeding Stuffs Act 1976. (London: HMSO)
5.   Radioactive Substances Act 1960 (8 & 9 Eliz. 2 CH 34) (London: HMSO)
6.   Health and Safety at Work etc. Act 1974 (C37) (London: HMSO)

7.   Consumer Protection Act 1961 (9 and 10 Eliz. 2 CH 40)
      (London: HMSO)
8.   DHSS Committee on Toxicity of Chemicals in Food, Consumer
      Products and the Environment (1982). Guidelines for the
      Testing of Chemicals for Toxicity. Report on Health and
      Social Subjects No. 27. (London: HMSO)
9.   DHSS Committee on Carcinogenicity of Chemicals in Food,
      Consumer Products and the Environment (1982). Guidelines
      for the Testing of Chemicals for Carcinogenicity. Report on
      Health and Social Subjects No. 25. (London: HMSO)
10.   DHSS Committee on Mutagenicity of Chemicals in Food, Con-
      sumer Products and the Environment (1981). Guidelines for
      the Testing of Chemicals for Mutagenicity. Report on Health
      and Social Subjects No. 24. (London: HMSO)
11.   Memorandum on The Testing of Novel Foods (1985).
      Guidelines for Testing. (London: Ministry of Agriculture,
      Fisheries and Food)
12.   Bunyan, PJ, Coomes, TJ and Elton, GAH (1984). Fundamen-
      tal and Applied Toxicology, 4, S263-77
13.   Medicines Act 1968. 1984 Guidance Notes on Applications for
      Product Licences, Department of Health and Social
      Security.(London: HMSO)
14.   Environmental Health, Anti-oxidants (1983). On the State of
      the Public Health for the Year 1982, 38 (London: HMSO)
15.   Goldberg, L (1982). The next 25 years in toxicology.
      Safety Evaluation and Regulation of Chemicals, 1st Interna-
      tional Conference, pp. 193-9. (Basel: Karger)
16.   Population Projections 1981-2001 (1984). Office of Population
      Censuses and Surveys, Series PP3, No. 5 (London: HMSO)
17.   Dukes, MN (1984). The Effects of Drug Regulation.
      (WHO)(Lancaster: MTP Press)
18.   Cromie, B (1979). Present problems: the effects of British
      regulations. Medicines for the Year 2000, 76. (London: Of-
      fice of Health Economics)
19.   Brimblecombe, RW and Dayan, AD (1985). Preclinical
      toxicity testing. Pharmaceutical Medicine, p. 36. (London:
      Edward Arnold)
20.   Rondel, RK (1985). The regulation of medicines in Europe.
      Pharmaceutical Medicine, p. 168. (London: Edward Arnold)
21.   Colin Jones, DG, Langman, MJS, Lawson, DH and Vessey,
      MP (1985). Post-marketing surveillance of the safety of
      cimetidine: twelve-month morbidity report. Q J Med, 54,
      215, 253

2
Toxicity Testing: Views of Animal Welfare Organizations

J. REMFRY

LOOK AHEAD

A question in an examination paper for an Honours Degree in Animal Welfare Studies in the 1990s could read: "Changes in the use of animals in toxicity testing in the 1980s were due more to pressure from the animal welfare organizations than to availability of new technology: discuss". The diligent student could recount the development of technologies based on cell, tissue and organ cultures, the use of computers and the means available to reduce animal numbers and to set less severe end-points. But he would then surely enlarge with enthusiasm on the building-up of public opinion against animal use, and the ways the governments of the time responded by enacting new legislation.

The more enterprising students might, if time permitted, digress on the ambivalent attitudes of most members of the public in the 1970s and 1980s, some of whom were quite vocal in demanding simultaneously safe consumer products and the protection of laboratory animals from pain, without being aware of the difficulties which still existed at that time in reconciling the two.

PUBLIC CONCERN ABOUT LABORATORY ANIMALS

Why has the public become so much more concerned about the use of animals in laboratories in the 1980s? There is no evidence to suggest that experiments are more painful, nor that the housing conditions of the animals have deteriorated, nor that more stolen pets are used in the laboratory. In fact the number of potentially painful experiments reported to the Home Office has declined steadily from about 5.5 million in 1976 to under 3.5 million in 1984[1]. The explanation appears to lie elsewhere. For example:

1. Better information. The old-established anti-vivisectionist societies have become more active in campaigning, and give their   subscribers more up-to-date information, including

27

photos of current situations, sometimes obtained by illegal entry into laboratories. These pictures can be unsettling. Biologists seeing them will probably look about their own departments with greater interest.

2. <u>Expectations about alternatives</u>. Publicity from some societies has led the public into an expectation that animals will soon be obsolete in laboratories. Smyth[2], in his invaluable review of alternative techniques, tried to explain why this was not so, and a meeting organized by FRAME in 1982 showed the current limitations of replacement techniques[3], but the message may be too unpalatable to be well received.

3. <u>Disillusionment with modern medicine</u>. In spite of all the animals that have died in the interests of medical research, people still fall ill, often with diseases such as cancer for which science cannot find a quick cure. This has led to some frustation and disillusionment with modern medicine, and a hope that alternative forms may offer greater relief without requiring the sacrifice of animals.

4. <u>Disillusionment with modern science</u>. Science has been blamed by some people for many of the ills of modern society, and these people sometimes view biologists as reckless users of animals, driven by curiosity into areas where they have no right to be.

5. <u>Environmental links</u>. Greater awareness of environmental problems, the scarcity of world food resources and the advantages of vegetarianism are often linked to a concern about the exploitation of animals, particularly laboratory animals.

6. <u>Animal rights</u>. Singer's book "Animal Liberation"[4] started a trend in philosophy in which the moral status of animals became a legitimate object of critical study. If slaves can be recognized as having the right to life and liberty, why not women? And if women, why not animals? On what basis does man justify the exploitation of animals? This thinking has affected the views of many rational people and might partly explain the increase in vegetarianism. However, young activists have taken this philosophy into areas of civil disobedience and even criminal damage not intended by the original authors, and have incurred the anger of many. As "The Times" leader said: "Man's inhumanity to animals is a focus of contemporary anarchy. Animal "liberation" and animal "rights" are so intoxicating a cause that some of those in its service believe themselves to be absolved from normal obligations of society and the law. They trespass, do criminal damage and threaten or endanger persons of whose lawful activities they disapprove, all without losing the sense of their own virtue. It is one of those causes that induce in enthusiasts the loss of all sense of proportion[5]".

Nevertheless, the idea of animals having innate rights which man has no right to take away has spread, so that, for example, it is now considered inappropriate in some schools for biology students to dissect animals.

VIEWS OF ANIMAL WELFARE ORGANIZATIONS

The animal welfare organizations may be divided into three categories. First, there are the societies involved in the practical protection of animals, through rescue, shelters and clinics. Then there are the animal welfare societies, such as UFAW, that are concerned with promoting the welfare of animals and with reforming the way society deals with animals. Third there are the organizations which seek radical changes in the law and society by, for example the abolition of vivisection. These organizations often embrace the animal rights philosophy.

Animal protection societies

The traditional animal welfare and protection societies such as those which rescue or re-home domesticated animals are unlikely to have a policy on toxicity testing. They may deplore any distress caused to animals in the laboratory, but their need for effective veterinary medicines and vaccines will be over-riding. Wildlife societies are more likely to be concerned about the indiscriminate use of agricultural poisons.

Royal Society for the Prevention of Cruelty to Animals

The RSPCA - in addition to its traditional work through its inspectors, clinics and homes - tries to influence the opinions of its members on a range of animal welfare topics, including animal experimentation. Their "Policy on Animal Experimentation"[6] states: "The RSPCA is opposed to all animal experiments or procedures which cause pain, suffering or distress." "The Society is also opposed to the use of animals in the testing of inessential substances such as cosmetics." The RSPCA advises its members to think carefully about the medicines and household products they buy, to avoid the inessential ones and to choose those that have been on the market a long time and so are less likely to be subject to tests on animals.

The Universities Federation for Animal Welfare

UFAW has always taken a particular interest in laboratory animals. The first edition of the "UFAW Handbook on the Care and Management of Laboratory Animals"[7] was, in 1947, a pioneering work, for the first time bringing together knowledge on how best to care for a wide range of animals. Another influential book commissioned by UFAW and published in 1959 was Russell and Burch's "The Principles of Humane Experimental Technique"[8]. It was here that the principle of the 3 Rs was first expounded. The 3 Rs: Replacement, Reduction and Refinement, is a shorthand categorization of the way scientists should plan their work in order to eliminate unnecessary suffering in laboratory animals. **Replacement** means the use of non-sentient material instead of living animals where possible. **Reduction** means designing experiments and selecting healthy animals so that the number needed to obtain a statistically significant result is the minimum. **Refinement** means selecting and perfecting the techniques involved so that trauma is reduced to a minimum. In the 20 years since publication, the idea of the 3 Rs has been welcomed and disseminated by many scientists as well as animal welfare organizations, all over the world, and has been applied to the questions of toxicity testing with beneficial results.

In the 1960s UFAW commissioned A. C. Frazer of the University of Birmingham to study the ways in which animals were used in the laboratory, particularly in toxicity testing. His results were presented at a UFAW symposium in 1969[9]. He stressed how important it was to choose the species of experimental animal carefully, selecting it on a basis of similarity of metabolism with the target species. He suggested that in acute toxicity studies, information gained on the effect of the test substances on possible target organs at various dose levels was more valuable than a precise LD-50 value, and also uses fewer animals. He also showed the beneficial effects of using disease-free animals in long-term studies.

These ideas were followed up in the 1972 symposium[10]. Here Mary Dawson, who was later to carry out research for UFAW, explained the limitations of tissue cultures in biomedical research. Walter Scott, then the Director of UFAW, expressed the view that the LD-50 test, while necessary for medicines with a narrow therapeutic margin, should not be used for relatively safe products such as cosmetics and soaps; national regulations should be looked at carefully to ensure that LD-50 values were never demanded unnecessarily.

UFAW gave evidence along these lines to the Home Office Committee of Enquiry into the LD-50 test under the chairmanship of Lord Cross. This Committee reported in 1979 and concluded that the LD-50 test must cause appreciable pain to a proportion of the animals subjected to them. It recommended that the test be allowed to continue, but "those who prescribe them or carry them out should always bear in mind that for "safety evaluation" purposes a degree of precision which calls for the use of a large number of animals is not necessary" and "wherever practicable a limit test should be used in preference to an LD-50"[11].

The Fund for the Replacement of Animals in Medical Experimentation (FRAME)

FRAME was founded in 1969 with its aim clearly stated in its title. It did not regard itself primarily as an animal welfare society, since it hoped to have nothing to do with animals. Under a succession of scientific directors, FRAME put forward ideas on the value of in vitro systems, lower organisms, computer simulation and other methods which had considerable influence on public attitudes[12]. Its policy altered under the direction of Michael Balls, who saw that Reduction and Refinement were important short term measures while working towards the ultimate goal of Replacement. He agreed with Smyth[2] and Rowan[13] that the term "alternative" should be redefined to include any method which reduces the numbers of animals required to achieve a comparable result, or which by refinement of techniques reduced the pain or suffering caused to the animals.

FRAME's ideas, like those of UFAW, have been widely used by other animal welfare societies and so have had a spreading influence amongst non-scientists. A factor in this process has been the Committee for Information on Animals in Research whose Information Sheets, primarily written for legislations, have also been distributed to animal welfare societies and have helped to focus their attention on particular issues[14].

Other organizations

As well as the older animal protection and welfare societies there are many new ones. Some of them are concerned with animal rights and campaign for the abolition of particular uses of animals. If their purpose is to change legislation they do not have charitable status.

The anti-vivisectionist societies are strictly speaking against any use of animals in the laboratory, but in recent years they have campaigned against the LD-50 and the Draize eye test as being particularly unacceptable to animal-lovers.

A number of societies have set up separate trusts to fund research which does not involve live animals, in order to speed up the process of replacement of animals by other systems. The best-known are probably the Dr Hadwen Trust, the Lawson Tait and Humane Research Trust and the Lord Dowding Fund.

PUTTING ANIMALS INTO POLITICS

The centenary of the Cruelty to Animals Act 1876 came and went without any promise for the government to introduce new legislation to protect laboratory animals. Lord Houghton of Sowerby decided that the time had come to "stop pussy-footing and start campaigning"[15]. He and the Director of the Scottish Society for the Prevention of Vivisection, Clive Hollands (who describes the campaign in "Compassion is the Bugler")[16], set up five joint consultative bodies of which one was the Committee for the Reform of Animal Experimentation (CRAE) in 1977. In 1978 these joined forces as the General Election Co-ordinating Committee for Animal Protection. CRAE's position was ambivalent. It was composed mainly of anti-vivisection societies, and yet it campaigned for reform, not abolition, of animal experimentation. For example, it demanded that "A determined effort should be made to restrict the use of animals in procedures which are not strictly for therapeutic purposes, e.g. the testing of cosmetics and toiletries, the testing of weapons and behavioural research". This campaign had little effect on voting patterns, but within the next few years two private members' bills were introduced to replace the Cruelty to Animals Act. Both failed.

Meanwhile CRAE, still under the secretaryship of Hollands,

31

had shed the British Union for the Abolition of Vivisection and the National Anti Vivisection Society and formed an alliance with the British Veterinary Association (BVA) and FRAME. Together, they submitted proposals[17] to the Home Office for new legislation which, while recognizing the necessity for toxicity testing, suggested methods of constraining it through licensing of procedures, limitation of the degree of pain to be inflicted and Codes of Practice.

In 1983 and 1985 the government published White Papers[18,19] setting out their proposals for new legislation. Many of the BVA-CRAE-FRAME suggestions had been incorporated. A number of anti-vivisection societies responded angrily to both Hollands and the Home Office and formed themselves into Mobilization for Laboratory animals against the Government's Proposals[20]. They demanded that any new legislation must include, as a basic minimum,

- a ban on cosmetic, tobacco and alcohol experiments;
- a ban on the Draize eye irritancy test;
- a ban on the LD-50 poisoning test;
- a ban on behavioural/psychological experiments;
- a ban on warfare experiments;
- a reconstitution of the Home Secretary's Advisory Committee on Animal Experiments, to exclude those who have a vested interest in the continuation of animal experiments.

Thus some of the issues raised more genteelly by the animal welfare organizations, and by scientists themselves, over the past 15 years, had now been projected as demands by the anti-vivisectionists. No government has yielded to such demands in the past, and is not likely to now, particularly since the present demands followed personal attacks and abuse to the responsible Minister at the Home Office. However, the regulatory bodies, which decide the data required for registration and marketing of, for example, medicines, have been responsive to requests from scientists for more flexible rules, particularly in the area of toxicity testing. This will make it possible for the government to discourage painful tests, so long as international harmonization of the regulations can be achieved.

PRESENT ISSUES

1. The lethal dose 50 test

As already described, the LD-50 has been under attack since the late 1960s. The objections to the test are that its sole purpose is to discover the lethal dose; that no analgesic may be given if the animal is in pain, and that the LD-50 value, however precisely calculated for an experimental animal, may be quite different in man.

At a meeting held by FRAME in 1982 their independent Toxicity Committee recommended that the LD-50 test should be discontinued for the testing of pharmaceuticals and most other chemicals and be replaced by more relevant studies. Not one of the delegates at the meeting (mostly toxicologists) wished to retain the LD-50 test in its classic form[3]. The British Toxicology Society supported this position and in 1984 published the Report of its Working Party on Toxicity[21]. They made specific recommendations for changes in the regulations for toxicity testing. Most notable was their suggestion that instead of test substances being given an LD-50 value they should be classified as Very Toxic, Toxic, Harmful or Unclassified. This would require far fewer animals and be quite sufficient for most chemicals.

In 1985 a petition against the LD-50 test carrying 500,000 signatures was presented to the House of Commons by Mr Roland Boyes, MP. The Home Secretary responded by welcoming the growing recognition by scientists and regulatory bodies that the test was increasingly unnecessary and pledging that, under the new system of control he was proposing, LD-50 tests would be used only when they were clearly justified. At about the same time the Medicines Commission announced that the LD-50 test would no longer be required for testing the antibiotic dactinomycin.

In the USA scientists had also been trying to reduce the numbers of animals used to obtain LD-50 values in safety testing. The regulatory authorities were forced to catch up with them when Henry Spira's Coalition to Abolish the LD-50 began campaigning in the early 1980s. By 1984 the Food and Drug Administration had reviewed its policy and decided that a statistically precise LD-50 was not required. In the same year the Environmental Protection Agency produced new guidelines aimed to reduce the number of animals killed in testing new chemicals. These guidelines suggest that 10 animals should normally be enough to determine the lethal dose.

So the classical LD-50 test, requiring up to 40 animals for its determination by any route, will soon be back where it belongs - the assay of medicinal substances with a narrow therapeutic margin. This is a success story for animal welfare in the UK and in the USA, but carries fewer lessons than the story of the Draize test.

2. Draize eye irritancy test

In 1948 some British scientists studying the effect of chemical warfare agents on the eyes of rabbits, reported:

> If a large drop [of mustard gas] be placed on the cornea and the eye allowed to close, a generalized lesion of great severity is produced..... For the first nine days the eyelids and ocular and palpebral conjunctiva are so swollen and oedematous that it is impossible to see the cornea. There is copious discharge which glues the lids together and mats the fur and causes it to fall out over a wide area around the eye.....[22].

It is doubtful whether such an experiment would be permitted to proceed beyond the initial damage in the UK now, even in a national emergency. Nevertheless, considerable damage to the conjunctiva and cornea may still occur in eye irritancy tests such as the Draize.

In 1978 Professor Smyth in his review of alternatives to animal experiments drew particular attention to the Draize eye test[2]. He suggested that, since it was widely used in the testing of cosmetics and shampoos, and since there was a possibility of considerable pain being caused to rabbits thereby, a major attempt was needed to find an alternative to the test. He pointed out that unlike general toxicity, involving many possible target sites, the Draize test was concerned only with the effect of the test substance on the epithelium and the cornea, and was thus a circumscribed problem.

Several laboratories in the UK and overseas took up the challenge, for example by using eyes removed from freshly killed rabbits[23]. The anti-vivisectionists used pictures of rabbits and descriptions of techniques in their literature.

Henry Spira, in "Fighting to Win", tells how he also took up the challenge, recognizing the Draize eye test as a single, significant injustice to animals and its abolition as a clearly limited and attainable goal. He used the US Freedom of Information Act to obtain the reports submitted by cosmetic companies on the safety testing of their products to the US Department of Agriculture. Pinpointing Revlon as the market leader he suggested they put $200,000 into developing non-animal tests, to replace the rabbits in the Draize eye test. Nothing happened, so Spira brought together 407 animal rights and animal protection organizations to form a Coalition to Abolish the Draize Test. They initiated an advertizing campaign showing a white rabbit with sticking plasters over its eyes, and invited readers to write to the president of Revlon stating that they would not use Revlon products until the company funded a research programme to develop alternatives.

Early in 1981 Revlon offered an annual grant of $250,000 to Rockefeller University to support work on in vitro cytotoxicity assays[25]. Then Avon put up the money for the Center of Alternatives to Animal Testing at Johns Hopkins University. This Center is now funded by several companies, trade associations and foundations, and is working on several fronts. Their "Newsletter"[26] describes two Draize-alternative projects, one using rabbit eye cells and the other human eye cells grown in vitro.

The success of these projects will not be known until the proposed new methods have been validated - that is, they have been compared with animal tests to see how accurately they can predict the damage done to the living eye by harmful substances. However, in the meantime the new methods can be used for pre-screening - that is for making rough estimates of the irritancy of substances suspected of being harmful. Many such tests were described at a meeting in Switzerland in 1984[27].

3. Pain

The LD-50 test and the Draize eye irritancy test were clear targets; but many other tests carry the risk of inflicting some pain or suffering on the animals involved. It is, after all, because of this that animal welfare societies worry about and anti-vivisectionist societies try to abolish animal experiments.

In 1962 UFAW held a symposium to review the current state of knowledge about pain in animals, and it was generally agreed that if an animal looks as if it is in pain, then we should give it the benefit of the doubt and assume that it is conscious of pain[28]. Little progress was made for several years, but then the discovery of endogenously produced morphine-like substances, the development of animal behavioural science and the availability of new powerful synthetic analgesics opened up the field so that the age-old question of pain could be examined afresh. The present state of knowledge was reviewed for UFAW by Iggo in 1984[29].

Veterinary surgeons who started to give their patients analgesics for the relief of postoperative pain were often surprised at the changes in behaviour they observed. Depression and reluctance to move, which had been regarded as normal postoperative behaviour, were now recognized as being largely a response to postoperative pain. Powerful analgesics of both the morphine and non-morphine type are now available for rodents as well as the larger animals, so there is little excuse for withholding them. For a review of the available drugs and recommended dosages see Flecknell[30].

Scientists are rarely trained in the detection or assessment of pain in experimental animals. Even veterinary surgeons who find it easy to recognize pain in farm and companion animals may find it difficult in wild ones such as Old World primates or in small rodents. Several groups are now working on the signs which should be looked for in different species. A scheme has been published by Morton and Griffiths which helps in the assessment of degrees of pain and gives guidance on when analgesics should be given or the experiment terminated[31].

The objective of legislation controlling animal experimentation must be to limit the amount of pain which a scientist is permitted to inflict on animals. To be effective the definition of pain must include forms of suffering such as hunger, thirst, disease and anxiety. The law must control not only the pain inflicted as a direct result of the licensed procedure but also any caused accidentally or by negligence.

In 1983 the RSPCA reviewed the control of animal experiments in the UK. Their Report on Pain and Suffering in Experimental Animals in the UK is available from the RSPCA in a shortened version[32]. Their Animal Experimentation Committee searched the learned journals and selected 35 papers from British laboratories published in the years 1976-1981 inclusive. They found little evidence of severe pain - not surprisingly, since it is unlikely to be admitted by an author in any part of the world, and in Britain would alert the Home Office to possible infringement of the law. However, they did find evidence of wasteful use of animals caused by poor experimental design, and to pain and suffering attributable to poor experimental technique and lack of postoperative analgesia. In some cases it was difficult to see the scientific justification for carrying out the painful procedure.

The Report was presented to the Home Secretary to consider while proposals for new legislation were being prepared. Although no formal acknowledgement was ever made to the RSPCA, the proposals in the White Papers published in 1983[18] and 1985[19] would have the effect of tightening up rules on pain and would also suggest that any painful procedure planned should be justifiable in terms of the scientific or medical merit of the project. Another proposal was that guidelines or a code of practice should be prepared to explain to licensees how the rules on pain should be applied.

In fact, similar guidelines are, at the time this book goes to press, already being prepared for publication by the Royal Society and UFAW; these are being written for scientists by scientists, to show what welfare standards can and should be achieved using present knowledge and drugs.

Even all these proposals do not solve the problem of pain caused to animals through ignorance or lack of experience. The key to this is surely training in the handling and use of animals; fortunately training courses are being encouraged by the Home Office and by employers and a published syllabus is available[33].

4. Alternatives to living animals

Pressure for the discovery, development and validation of new replacement techniques for animals is coming from scientists, industry and the animal welfare organizations.

Cell biology is a thriving field and some of the fundamental work is bound to lead to methods which can be developed as alternatives to living animals. The pharmaceutical, chemical and cosmetics industries have the incentive to develop in vitro tests as a matter of convenience and to counter the rising costs of work with animals. The charities raising money for research into alternatives are still well-supported; because of the desperate need for funds in the universities, these charities are now able to be more selective about the projects they support. "ATLA" published by FRAME, has helped to spread knowledge of good new techniques[12]. The role of government seems to be to run along behind. Since the late 1970s the Home Office has exhorted its licensees to use non-animal alternatives wherever possible, but the government did litle in real terms to encourage the development of alternatives, and they really cannot take the credit for the falling numbers of animals used each year. The numbers used in the pharmaceutical and related industries has indeed fallen, but so has the number of new products brought to market.

In 1984 the UK government took an unprecedented step in offering FRAME £50,000 p.a. for 3 years to carry out three projects: to develop the use of human tissue culture; to validate some existing in vitro tests in order to reduce the number of animals used in toxicity testing, and to make information on tissue culture techniques more widely available to scientists. This has been greeted as a positive and welcome step by scientists, politicians and the public.

In the USA the government has put no money into developing

new alternative methods, but in late 1983 the Congressional Office of Technology Assessment (OTA) did set up an 18-month study on laboratory animal alternatives. A panel was formed including animal welfare representatives and scientists, and they were asked to examine the current pattern of animal use in toxicity testing and other fields; to assess how animal usage could be reduced; and to look at the advantages of in vitro tests. Their recommendations are not yet published, but are expected to lead to a wider interest in "alternatives".

It does indeed seem that now, in the mid-1980s the scene is set for the use of non-sentient alternatives to start making a genuine contribution to the fall in numbers of animals used in potentially painful tests.

THE FUTURE

There are many issues outstanding which need more attention if animal usage is to be reduced and procedures are to be less severe. For example:

(a) Current methods for the production and testing of certain vaccines need to be changed. The scientists and regulatory bodies involved are well aware of this, as a meeting in 1985 of the International Association of Biological Standardization showed[34].

(b) Duplication of animal tests may result from the refusal of companies to share data. A system which ensures confidentiality could surely be devised.

(c) Animal tests now considered unnecessary in an exporting country may still be carried out in order to satisfy the requirements of an importing country. The proposed European Convention for the Protection of Vertebrate Animals used for Experimental and Other Scientific Purposes contains a part on recognition of procedures carried out in the territory of another contracting party. Article 29 proposes that unnecessary repetition of safety tests should be prevented by each nation recognizing the results of procedures carried out in another contracting nation. Also they should help each other by sharing information on the procedures carried out. Discussions within Europe will be necessary to ensure that the spirit of these proposals is included in new national laws within the member countries of the Council of Europe. Further discussions will be needed to include the non-European nations. It will probably not be easy.

(d) A significant reduction in the numbers of animals required for particular tests has already been achieved by improving the quality of the animals used. More needs to be done to improve and specify the health and genetic status of animals, and to increase comparability of results by specifying caging and environmental conditions which are known to be optimal.

UFAW has been co-operating with the Laboratory Animal Science Association in this field[35].

Laboratory animal science has been greatly under-funded in the UK since the Medical Research council closed down its Laboratory Animal Centre in 1981[36]. It is hardly the place of the animal welfare societies to make good this deficit, but there are a few which can co-operate with other bodies to do basic work. In 1984 UFAW was commissioned by the Home Office to carry out a study on how cage conditions for laboratory rats could be improved; it is now under way in the University of London. This gesture from the government, while welcome, is not likely to satisfy the increasing public and scientific concern for the welfare of animals inside laboratories and animal houses.

(e) The public is expecting greater accountability from scientists on their use of animals. Some scientists protest they are already fully accountable to the bodies which fund their work and their colleagues and, through their publications, to the world at large[37]. Others appreciate that this does not satisfy the public. In Sweden, scientists wishing to perform painful procedures must submit their proposals to a local ethical committee on which non scientist members of the community are represented[38]. In the USA, Institutional Animal Care and Use Committees have community repre-sentation[39]. In Switzerland, biomedical workers are urged to comply with a set of published ethical principles as well as being subject to legal control[40]. The concept of research review committees which include ethical considerations in their remit is being encouraged by a number of animal welfare organizations; for a review, see Britt[41]. Also, for those countries considering some sort of legal control over animal experiments, the Council for International Organizations of Medical Science has proposed some Guiding Principles for Biomedical Research involving Animals[42].

Peer review systems, codes of practice and guidelines will be proliferating in the late 1980s as Standard Operating Procedures did in the early 1980s. However, all this will still not satisfy some sections of the public, because there is still secrecy surrounding what actually goes on inside laboratories. This secrecy is increasing as security is tightened against the day when the Animal Liberation Front pays a visit. How should the public be informed of what is being carried out on their behalf? At present the unfortunate truth is that some newspapers are still more likely to publish shock-horror stories of a goat with a transplanted udder than with explanations of how animal research has contributed to advances in transplant surgery. The Research Defence Society has produced some useful leaflets[41], but a major educational programme is required, undertaken by a neutral body to avoid the accusation of bias.

Campaigning in the UK

The guerrilla tactics of the Animal Liberation Front have spread from the UK to other parts of the western world, including North America. In return it may be expected that activist organizations in the UK will try to adopt the campaigning methods so successfully used in the USA. Attempts to form groupings similar to the US coalitions have failed so far, probably because none has yet focused on a single vulnerable issue. Even in the US the coalitions break up, and the separate organizations continue the campaigns on their own, in order to maintain their own identities.

For example, the Humane Society of the United States has followed up the Draize eye test campaign with its own all-out offensive against cosmetic testing on animals[42]. They claim that "cruel" testing could be stopped immediately if consumers demanded it. This claim would indeed be true if consumers refused to buy innovative products containing "miracle" ingredients and if they were prepared to accept batch testing by unvalidated methods. In fact some in vitro methods could probably be validated remarkably quickly if the consumer pressure were strong enough. It is too early yet to judge the success of this offensive.

In the UK no such radical approach has yet been seriously attempted. Beauty Without Cruelty and other similar but smaller organizations encourage their members to use cosmetics containing ingredients which have been neither derived from nor tested on animals. Such cosmetics are expensive and are not available in High Street shops. Building up a consumer lobby powerful enough to influence the large cosmetic manufacturers would require time, skill and resources, but it is within the realm of possibilities. Many consumer and single-issue groups are learning to organize themselves and realize their potential power. What would be needed in this case is a law requiring labelling of goods with a full listing of the ingredients, combined with an educational campaign to explain to consumers the implications for animal welfare of the various ingredients - their source and how they are developed and tested. If the consumers chose their purchases accordingly, the market would soon be affected. An animal welfare coalition could help to launch such a campaign.

Coalitions formed for a specific purpose will naturally tend to break up once the objective has been achieved. They may break up earlier, if there is disagreement over the exact end-point to be aimed for, e.g. whether it is the partial or total abolition of the targeted procedure.

Coalitions could have unwanted effects. Manufacturers faced with a powerful coalition may be stampeded into making rash or misleading claims about the reduced role of animals in their laboratories. More seriously, manufacturers and governments might be frightened into making genuine concessions which they think will satisfy the coalitions, only to find that the more extreme members regard that step as a minor one in their overall plan, and use the concession to force new ones. This could lead to the elimination of testing procedures using animals which are still actually required for the safety of the public; or to animal research being made so expensive in the UK that laboratories are forced to transfer overseas.

CONCLUSION

By 1990 there will be new techniques available in toxicology and many non-animal tests will have been validated. In medical research there will probably be greater use of epidemiological information, clinical material and human volunteers. It will probably be the scientists more than the animal welfare organizations, and perhaps particularly those scientists who are also members of animal welfare organizations, who will be working most effectively to overthrow the last vestiges of conservatism amongst the professors, industrialists and regulatory bodies. The way will then be open for real changes in legislation and a significant reduction in the use of animals in painful procedures.

When this real reduction has been achieved, everybody will congratulate themselves and take the credit for their own interest group. Only students of the subject will seriously analyse whether the animal welfare interests had co-operated with each other enough to constitute an effective animal welfare lobby and, if so, whether the animal welfare lobby had pushed the scientists or whether the scientists had led the lobby.

In the meantime, new horizons will have appeared to take the attention of the animal welfare organizations: genetic engineering, the use of animals in space and other problems so far undreamed of

REFERENCES

1. Home Office (1985). Statistics of Experiments on Living Animals, Great Britain, 1984. (London: HMSO; Cmnd 9574)
2. Smyth, DH (1978). Alternatives to Animal Experiments. (London: Scolar Press in association with The Research Defence Society)
3. Balls, M, Riddell, RJ and Worden, A (eds) (1983). Animals and Alternatives in Toxicity Testing. (London: Academic Press)
4. Singer, P (1976). Animal Liberation: a New Ethics for Our Treatment of Animals. (London: Jonathan Cape)
5. Editorial (1985). The Times, 16 May
6. Royal Society for the Prevention of Cruelty to Animals (1984). Policy on Animal Experimentation. (Horsham, West Sussex: RSPCA) See also leaflet: Animal Experimentation
7. Worden, AN (ed.) (1947). UFAW Handbook on the Care and Management of Laboratory Animals, (London: Bailliere, Tindall & Cox; 6th edn. (1986) (in press). (London: Longmans)
8. Russell, WMS and Burch, RL (1959). The Principles of Humane Experimental Technique. (London: Metheun)
9. Universities Federation for Animal Welfare (1969). The Use of Animals in Toxicological Studies. (Potters Bar, Herts.: UFAW)
10. Universities Federation for Animal Welfare (1972). The Rational Use of Living Systems in Bio-medical Research. (Potters Bar, Herts.: UFAW)
11. Cross, G (Chairman) (1979). Report on the LD-50 test presented to the Secretary of State by the Advisory Com-

mittee on the administration of the Cruelty to Animals Act 1876. (London: Home Office)

12. ATLA. Alternatives to Animals. Published four times a year by FRAME, Nottingham

13. Rowan, AN (1984). Of Mice, Models, & Men: a Critical Evaluation of Animal Research. (Albany: State University of New York Press)

14. Committee for Information on Animal Research. Information Sheets 1-20, published 1977-1985. List available from 9D Stanhope Road, London N6 5HE

15. Houghton, Lord (1979). Animals and the law: moral and political issues. In Paterson, D and Ryder RD (eds) Animals' Rights: a Symposium. (London: Centaur Press for the RSPCA)

16. Hollands, C (1980). Compassion is the Bugler: the Struggle for Animal Rights. (Edinburgh: Macdonald)

17. British Veterinary Association, Committee for the Reform of Animal Experimentation and Fund for the Replacement of Animals in Medical Experiments (1983). Animal Experimentation in the UK - proposals submitted to the Home Secretary jointly by BVA, CRAE and FRAME, c/o 10 Queensferry Street, Edinburgh

18. Home Office (1983). Scientific Procedures on Living Animals. (London: HMSO, Cmnd 8883)

19. Home Office (1985). Scientific Procedures on Living Animals. (London: HMSO Cmnd 9521)

20. Mobilization for Laboratory Animals against the Government's Proposals. (1983). Legislate to Liberate, c/o 51 Harley Street, London

21. British Toxicology Society Working Party on Toxicity (1984). Special Report: a new approach to the classification of substances and preparations on the basis of their acute toxicity. Human Toxicol, 3, 85-92

22. Mann, I, Pullinger, BD and Pirie, A (1948). An experimental and clinical study of the reaction of the anterior segment of the eye to chemical injury, with special reference to chemical warfare agents. Monograph of Br J Ophthalmol

23. Burton, ABG, York, M and Lawrence, RS (1981). The in vitro assessment of severe eye irritants. Food Cosmet Toxicol, 19

24. Spira, H (1985). Fighting to win. In Singer, P (ed.) In Defence of Animals. (Oxford: Blackwell)

25. Stark, DM and Shopsis, C (1983). Developing alternative assay systems for toxicity testing. In Role of Animals in Biomedical Research, 406. Annals of NY Acad Sci, 92-103

26. Push, S (ed.) The Johns Hopkins Centre for Alternatives to Animal Testing. Four issues per year. (Baltimore: Johns Hopkins School of Public Health)

27. Reinhardt, C, Bosshard, E and Schlatter, C (eds) (1985). Irritation testing of skin and mucous membranes. A special issue of Food and Chemical Toxicology, 23

28. Keele, CA and Smith R (1962). The Assessment of Pain in Man and Animals. (London: Universities Federation for Animal Welfare)

29. Iggo, A (1985). Pain in Animals. The 3rd Hume Memorial
     Lecture. (Potters Bar, Herts.: UFAW)
30. Flecknell, PA (1984). The relief of pain in laboratory
     animals. Lab Anim, 18, 147-60
31. Morton, DB and Griffiths, PHM (1985). Guidelines on the
     recognition of pain, distress and discomfort in experimental
     animals and an hypothesis for assessment. Vet Rec, 116,
     431-6
32. Royal Society for the Prevention of Cruelty to Animals
     (1983). Pain and Suffering in Experimental Animals in the
     UK - a report by the Animal Experimentation Advisory Com-
     mittee of the RSPCA. Available from RSPCA, Horsham, W.
     Sussex.
33. Smith, MW (Chairman) (1984). Report of the Working Party
     on courses for animal licensees. Lab Anim, 18, 209-20
34. International Association of Biological Standardization. Al-
     ternatives to the Use of Animals in the Development and Con-
     trol of Vaccines. (Geneva: IABS) (In press)
35. UFAW (1984). Standards in Laboratory Animal Management
     (Proceedings of a symposium organised by the Laboratory
     Animal Science Association and UFAW). (Potters Bar,
     Herts.: UFAW)
36. Remfry, Jenny (1985). Recent developments in laboratory
     animal science. In: Animal Experimentation; Improvements
     and Alternatives - Replacement Refinement and Reduction.
     Proceedings of a symposium. Published by FRAME as a
     supplement to ATLA
37. Briscoe, TJ (1984). The accountability of scientists. In:
     RDS Newsletter - Medical Progress for Men and Animals,
     July. (London: Research Defence Society)
38. Swedish Medical Research Council (1978 and 1982). The Use
     of Experimental Animals in Medical and Biological Research.
     English translation 1982. (Stockholm: Mediciniska
     Forskningsradet)
39. Institute of Laboratory Animal Resources, National Research
     Council (1985). Guide for the Care and Use of Laboratory
     Animals. (Bethesda, Md.: National Institutes of Health)
40. Weibel, ER (Chairman) (1984). Ethical Principles and
     Guidelines for Scientific Experiments on Animals. (Berne:
     Swiss Academy of Medical Sciences and Swiss Academy of
     Sciences)
41. Britt, DP (1985). Research Review (Ethical) Committees for
     Animal Experimentation. (Potters Bar, Herts.: UFAW)
     Research Defence Society. Are Animal Experiments Neces-
     sary for Cosmetic Products? and other leaflets undated.
     (London: Research Defence Society)
42. Council for International Organizations of Medical Sciences
     (1985). International Guiding Principles for Biomedical Re-
     search Involving Animals. (Geneva: CIOMS)
     Humane Society of the United States (1985). Close-up
     Report. February. (Washington DC: HSUS)

3

Risks in Medical Intervention: Balancing Therapeutic Risks and Benefits*

W. H. W. INMAN

INTRODUCTION

It has been estimated that about 100 billion human beings have walked on the surface of the Earth. If this is correct, it is an intriguing thought that one in 25 of them is alive today. In spite of famine, floods, plagues and wars, enough of each generation have survived not only to replace those lost in natural or self-inflicted disasters but also to expand the species at a rate which creates risks almost infinitely greater than any that we will discuss this evening. Our numbers have increased, we live much longer and we have more time to indulge in one of our favourite obsessions, which is concern about risk.

Since national vital statistics were first collected in 1840, mortality in the first year of life has fallen from one in seven born alive to one in 500, a reduction by a factor of 70. All other age groups have shown a large reduction, ranging from about twenty-fold in children to ten-fold in young and middle-aged adults, and to a more modest 50% in the elderly[1]. These statistics suggest that England has become a less risky place to live in. We can see the effects of improved hygiene and nutrition and of medical intervention in its widest sense. This success in risk reduction has been achieved by taking risks - mostly very small ones - for any kind of medical intervention involves some risk.

I shall concentrate on that part of medical intervention which we call **drug therapy**. During the quarter of a century in which I have been concerned with drug safety, about 7 billion drug prescriptions have been written by doctors in England, an average of about six per person per year. Doctors prescribe from a list of several thousand products, many of which produce great benefit at remarkably little risk. During these 25 years only one of them, thalidomide, has been responsible for an accident in this country

----

*A reprint of the Wolfson College Lecture, Oxford, 31 January 1984. Reprinted by kind permission of Oxford University Press

which could, by any stretch of the imagination, be termed a "disaster". The media, however, have inflated a number of small-scale incidents such as the "Opren" (benoxaprofen) affair to resemble thalidomide, and several drugs have recently been removed by the authorities on very questionable evidence.

Compared with the risks of smoking, drinking or travel, the risks involved in drug treatment are minute, yet they continue to provide ideas for the entertainment industry (the media), stories for journalists, votes for politicians and income for lawyers. The public have an undeniable right to be informed about the risks of drug treatment, but they also have a right to expect that the information presented to them is accurate and meaningful. Much of the information is heavily polluted with nonsense, but this is not always the journalist's fault. Twenty-three years after thalidomide we are shockingly incapable of providing even rough estimates of the risks or benefits of the drugs we prescribe, and we are inept at communicating what few statistics are available in a way which will inform people without alarming them.

My plan for this evening is to share some thoughts with you about the factors which affect our concept of risk, to suggest a simple way in which risk statistics could be made more palatable, to emphasize the difficulty we have in finding data on drug risks, and finally, to tell you something of the progress of a new method for postmarketing surveillance which we have developed in Southampton and which may help to fill some of the gaps in our knowledge.

WHAT DO WE MEAN BY RISKS AND BENEFITS

Risk is the **probability that something bad will happen**, and benefit the **probability that something good will happen**. Both risk and benefit must be expressed numerically[2]. Many people are uncomfortable about handling numbers, but, unless we come to grips with the problems of comparing the good and bad effects of medical intervention using numbers, we cannot hope to judge whether or not these risks are acceptable.

Usually we have to measure two levels of risk from treatment: firstly a small risk that a chosen treatment will occasionally kill or permanently disable the patient, and secondly a larger risk that it will cause temporary discomfort or inconvenience. I shall confine my discussion to the smaller risk since the common non-lethal side-effects and the proportion of people who will benefit from a drug are usually predicted during premarketing trials.

We also have to consider different types of risk/benefit situation, and there are perhaps four major types. When we are considering life-threatening disease we need to compare the risk that the patient will die from the disease with the risk of fatal complications of treatment. A more frequent and perhaps more difficult problem is where we have an effective treatment for a non-lethal disease which will, on rare occasions, produce a severe or fatal reaction. Here we have to decide how large a risk of death is acceptable in relation to the anticipated improvement in the quality of life. More difficult still is the treatment of a healthy person in order to prevent some naturally occurring phenomenon such as pregnancy or sea-sickness. Even more extreme is the treatment of an individual for the general benefit of others, as in whooping cough immunization, or for the benefit of those not yet conceived as in vaccination against German measles.

When considering the risk of death either from a disease or from the drugs used to treat it, we tend to think of these risks as one chance of dying per hundred, per thousand or per some other number. What we are actually saying is not that there is a risk of dying, since we all die, but that there is a risk that we will die **before our time**. In other words that there is a risk that we may suffer **loss of life expectancy**. Conversely, nobody can "save a life", only extend it.

It is not merely a question of lives lost or gained. We must always compare **time** lost or gained, not forgetting of course that quality may be more important than quantity. Our perception of risk may be very different if we have an expectation of 50 years than if we have only 5. Recent problems with anti-arthritic drugs have sharpened my concern about our perception of risk in the treatment of very elderly patients who have the shortest life expectancy and who are more likely to suffer adverse drug reactions than younger people. As I get older I think I might opt to trade some years for greater comfort and mobility. On the other hand the less there is to go the more I want to hang on to what is left because there is such a lot still to do and it is such fun doing it.

RISK PERCEPTION

Perception of risk is based on fear rather than statistics, and on the extent to which individuals identify with the various groups of risk-takers. Many factors influence our perception of risk. Obviously, if **large numbers** of accidents of a particular type occur, they are more interesting than a few isolated accidents. When a **large group** of people die in one accident, it may be reported as a disaster, while if the same number of individuals perish in separate accidents their deaths may not be noted. If four jumbo jets were to crash in England each week for several consecutive weeks, people would give up flying, but this is probably similar to the weekly toll from cigarette smoking. Accidents with an **acute onset** cause more alarm than those which have an insidious onset, cancer being an exception. **Unusual events** are more interesting than familiar ones. AIDS in homosexuals provides better copy for journalists than resistance to anti-malarials in the third world. It is hardly surprising that accidents in which **children** are the victims are more newsworthy than those affecting adults, or that damage caused by drugs used by **healthy people**, such as women using oral contraceptives, is more interesting than when sick patients are affected. An attack on a pop star or a president will be news for months or years, while you or I might merit only a few column inches in the local newspaper. If we choose to do something risky, like boxing or hang-gliding, we are willing to accept a much higher risk than when exposure to risk is **involuntary**, as in public transport. Most people believe that all drugs must be totally effective and totally safe, and if a possible **scapegoat** such as the manufacturer of a drug or officials who agreed to its marketing, can be identified, public indignation is aroused, champions of the alleged victims form "action groups", journalists rush half-considered facts to their sub-editors and attorneys in the US, hovering round the beds of the afflicted like septic poltergeists, vie with each other to establish new records in contingency fees[3].

COMPARISONS

If we are told that we have only a 50/50 chance of surviving an operation, we will have a fairly clear concept of its severity. Does it really make any difference, however, if a surgeon tells us that the risk of serious complications is one in a thousand or one in a million? A young woman may be scared stiff by the idea that the Pill could be associated with a risk of dying of one in 100,000, but if the same woman had some discomfort from gall stones and she was told the truth about the risks of surgery, which may be two orders of magnitude greater, she will probably not hesitate to go on the waiting list for the operation.

A few months ago I was exposed on television to an audience of general practitioners. They demanded that I should classify drug risks as acceptable or unacceptable. My reply was that I believed my job was to measure risks, to inform people and then to leave them to make up their own minds whether or not to take them. I was not arrogant enough to tell them whether or not these risks were acceptable in individual cases. Under pressure from the interviewer, one general practitioner suggested that she would be happy if the drugs which she was prescribing were "no more dangerous than aspirin", thus revealing instantly the awful truth that neither she nor I knew how dangerous aspirin might be.

I am very concerned about a recent trend in official judgements, on both sides of the Atlantic, which seems to be based on the **absolute** number of events that have been reported rather than on the **relative risks** in relation to other risks. To illustrate my concern: even though a serious event such as a report of one death from treating 100,000 patients may reflect only a very low risk, this is regarded important if the overall use of the drug is very large. In treating two million patients the total number of deaths each year would be 20. A figure of this magnitude would put the authorities under pressure to remove the drug because of the general view that public action should be taken on the basis of absolute numbers and not on the basis of relative risk. No-one would say that 20 deaths are not important, but I feel they really should be seen in relation to the two million benefited, otherwise the authorities will remove many drugs carrying a very low risk simply because they are used on a large scale, which in turn is because they are effective and therefore popular among patients and doctors. We will then find ourselves obliged to continue to use older remedies which may well be less effective and more dangerous. Officials must show more fortitude in dealing with public and political pressure whipped up by the story-tellers. It is easy to avoid criticism and may even seem praiseworthy to "ban the drug". It requires experience and courage to delay action until evidence has been assembled and the risks and benefits compared objectively.

In his Richard Dimbleby lecture of 1978, Lord Rothschild pointed out that "**Comparisons, far from being odious, are the best antidote to panic**"[4]. He went on to say that whenever anybody makes a statement about an accident or the number of people involved in it, he should always ask two simple questions.

1. "Is the risk stated in a straightforward language that I can understand, such as one in 1000? If not, why not?"

2. "Is the risk stated per year, per month, per day or per some period of time? If not, I shall ignore the information."

Few public statements by government agencies, politicians, pressure groups or journalists satisfy these two simple requirements. Let us look at a recent example.

In July 1982 the DHSS announced that the licence for the arthritis drug "Opren" (benoxaprofen) had been suspended. Information was given by officials to the press several days before the Committee on Safety of Medicines had had a chance to inform doctors, who should have been the first to know about the evidence behind this statement. It led to panic among patients, many of whom had found the drug to be effective, and anger among doctors. It increased fears about the safety of a whole group of drugs which, in my view, has led to unnecessarily harsh action against some of them.

Even when an attempt was made to explain the reasons behind the action, we were little better off. I quote from a letter to doctors and pharmacists dated 3 August 1982[5]:

> The Committee on Safety of Medicines has received over 3500 reports of adverse reactions associated with this drug; included among these reports are 61 fatal cases, predominantly in the elderly. Having regard to these reports there is concern about the serious toxic effects of the drug on various organ systems, particularly the gastro-intestinal tract, the liver and bone marrow, in addition to the known effects on the skin, eyes and nails.

The fact that most of the 3500 reports were of photosensitivity, which was a common side-effect of the drug, well known to have been a problem long before it was marketed, was not mentioned. More important, there was no mention of the size of the denominator with which the 3500 reports or the 61 deaths could be compared. Sales estimates are readily available, and it was known that more than half a million patients had been treated with the drug. True, the statement hinted that the main risk appeared to be in elderly people; this is true of many drugs, but there was no mention that this might have been due to accumulation of the drug because of its slower metabolism and excretion by elderly people, a fact which had been reported by the manufacturers at the 15th International Conference of Rheumatology in Paris in June 1981, one year before action was taken by the Licensing Authority[6]. Neither of Lord Rothschild's simple questions was answered. There was no indication of the size of the risk, nor of the time period during which the deaths had occurred. No comparisons were made which could have been an antidote to panic.

SCALE OF RISK

Let us see if we can think of a way in which the risks of diseases and drugs could be arranged on some sort of scale and presented in a way which would allow comparisons to be made.

Estimates of risk usually have very wide confidence limits and the majority are really guesstimates. More often than not the best we can do is to guess at the order of magnitude within which the risk falls. Because the range of risks is extremely wide, embracing many orders of magnitude, a logarithmic scale is convenient. So let us make a start with a logarithmic scale of risks of death per unit population per year (Table 3.1). Please note that the numerical value of the "risk level" is equal to the number of digits in the denominator. This makes it easy to remember the appropriate level, but has the disadvantage that the largest numbers are associated with the smallest risks. I have not yet found alternative words for "risk level" which would link the highest numbers with the perception of greatest safety.*

Table 3.1 Logarithmic scale of risk levels

Risk Level	Range	
1	1 in 1	- 1 in 9
2	1 in 10	- 1 in 99
3	1 in 100	- 1 in 999
4	1 in 1000	- 1 in 9999
5	1 in 10,000	- 1 in 99,999
6	1 in 100,000	- 1 in 999,999
7	1 in 1,000,000	- 1 in 9,999,999
8	1 in 10,000,000	- 1 in 99,999,999

*"Safety Index Number" is perhaps more satisfactory. I hesitated to suggest this because no drug can be completely safe.

In Table 3.2 I have arranged some examples of fatal conditions extracted from the Registrar General's mortality statistics for England and Wales for 1981. During that year about one in 86 people died and deaths from any cause thus fall in risk level 2. Cancer falls in level 3, peptic ulcer in level 4 and so on. The low risk for rheumatic fever is especially interesting. When I started to practise medicine, rheumatic fever was a major cause of morbidity and mortality, especially from heart disease. It has now virtually disappeared as a result of the **totally irresponsible use of antibiotics by general practitioners!** At least this is how many teachers of therapeutics, fearing the emergence of resistant strains of bacteria, viewed the routine use of antibiotics for sore throats and other minor infections. Perhaps, without realizing it, general practitioners have effectively wiped out a major cause of death and debility.

For comparison, in Table 3.3, I have shown the risk levels for violent or accidental deaths. Thanks to seat belts, motor vehicle traffic accidents have now fallen to level 5. Homicide lies in level 6 and so do aircraft accidents. The chances of being killed by lightning are less than one per 10 million (level 8), about the same as the combined risk of insect and snake bite and poisonous plants.

Table 3.2 Risk of death from certain diseases in England and Wales 1981

Risk level and deaths per year		Cause of death
1	1-	
2	10-	(any cause)
3	100-	Cancer, coronary disease, stroke
4	1000-	Peptic ulcer
5	10,000	Arthritis, asthma, cirrhosis, diabetes
6	100,000-	Pregnancy*, VD
7	1,000,000-	Tetanus, measles, whooping cough
8	10,000,000-	Acute rheumatic fever

*Females only.

The comparative figures for motor vehicle or aircraft accidents should, more realistically, be calculated for people who drive in motor cars or fly in aircraft, and should perhaps be expressed as the risk per so many journeys or thousands of miles travelled. Similarly, when we start to compare the risks of drugs with the risks of disease, we are interested, not so much in the death rate among the general population, as in the death rate in groups of patients suffering from the particular disease who need these drugs. In Table 3.4 I have firstly transcribed some of the details from Table 3.2 into a "general population" column, and secondly, created a column for "patients with specified disease", in which the risk level is that for mortality in groups of patients suffering from certain diseases. It can be seen that the risk of death, if you are suffering from a disease, is usually one or two orders of magnitude greater than the risk in the general population.

Table 3.3 Risk of violent or accidental death in England and Wales 1981

Risk level and deaths per year	Violent and accidental deaths
1 1-	
2 10-	
3 100-	
4 1000-	
5 10,000-	Motor vehicles, burns, falls, suicide
6 100,000-	Homicide, railways, aircraft
7 1,000,000-	Falling objects
8 10,000,000-	Lightning, animal and plant venom

In Table 3.5 I confine my attention to arthritis, firstly transcribing from Table 3.4 the risk level for a patient with that disease, and secondly estimating the probable risk of three drugs that have been regarded as "dangerous" and banned from use in general practice. Arthritis is not, as some people imagine, a non-lethal condition. I have placed the risk in level 3, but it could easily fall into level 2. Patients become immobile and suffer from infections and fractures, they undergo surgery with all its attendant risks and, when in severe pain, they have even been reported as suicides. I have put phenylbutazone at level 5, on the basis of a survey I conducted of all deaths from aplastic anaemia occurring in the country during 1976. I estimated the risk of death to be about one in 50,000 exposures (each exposure being, on average, of two months' duration)[7].

50

The deaths suspected to have been due to liver or kidney failure among patients taking "Opren" (benoxaprofen) reported to the Committee on Safety of Medicines (CSM) probably correspond to a death rate of the order of one in 25,000 (level 5). The reported incidence of fatal anaphylaxis due to "Zomax" (zomepirac) is one death per 2 million patients treated. This places this particular risk in level 7, hardly justifying removal from the market which followed a "trial by television" resulting from a single death reported in the USA. In making these comparisons we must remember that one unfortunate death of an elderly patient represents a few lost years of life while the removal of the drug may mean the loss of millions of years of more comfortable and more enjoyable life.

Table 3.4 Comparison of annual death rate in general population and in groups of patients suffering from certain diseases

Risk level	General population	Patients with specified diseases
1		Tetanus
2		Cancer, diabetes, peptic ulcer
3	Cancer	Arthritis
4	Peptic ulcer	
5	Arthritis, diabetes	Whooping cough
6		
7	Whooping cough, tetanus	
8		

The general point I am making is that even with those drugs which are actively under suspicion, the mortality during treatment is two or even more orders of magnitude, that is ten or one hundred, or even one thousand times **less** than the risk of dying from the disease. Unfortunately, time does not permit discussion of risks of other forms of treatment, such as treatment for hypertension or peptic ulcer, but almost every attempt I made to place a risk at the appropriate level resulted in a similar conclusion.

The idea of arranging estimates of risk on a logarithmic scale is not new. Heilmann and Urquhart proposed a risk scale based on what they termed "unicohorts", which are groups of people sharing some common diagnostic or demographic characteristics, such as all patients with diabetes or all women of childbearing age[8]. In their scheme, risks were expressed in "risk dilution units" on a "risk dilution scale" which is logarithmic. It is more sophisticated than mine and would take too long to describe this evening, but their conclusions were similar. The fact that a level of risk of treatment could be seen to be below the level of risk of the disease would, I believe, be clearly understood by the public. Repeated explanations that each level of risk actually represents a

Table 3.5 Risk of three drugs used in the treatment of arthritis

Risk level	Anti-arthritic drugs
1	
2	
3	Arthritis*
4	
5	Benoxaprofen - jaundice and renal failure
	Phenylbutazone - aplastic anaemia
6	
7	Zomepirac - anaphylaxis
8	

*It is possible that the incidence of fatal complications of arthritis exceeds 1 per 100 per year and that the true risk lies within level 2

frequency which is ten times less than the level above it, would help to defuse scare stories. Even if a risk had not been measured accurately, a statement of the probable risk level based on the available evidence would usually reassure rather than frighten people. If the predicted risk level was shown to lie too close to that of the disease to be acceptable for all patients, this method of presentation would help to justify a decision to limit its use to certain high-risk groups. When considering the treatment of conditions which carry a high risk of death (e.g. a disease in level 2), it might be acceptable to use a drug which carries a risk of death or serious adverse drug reaction which places it one or preferably two levels lower (correspondingly in level 3 or preferably 4). When considering conditions which are disabling but carry much lower risk of death (e.g. a disease in level 5). perhaps a two- or three-level separation would be preferred (correspondingly in level 7 or 8), though that implies knowledge of risk from drugs at extremely low levels, since level 8 is one in 10,000,000 to one in 99,999,999.

MORBIDITY AND MORTALITY ESTIMATES IN DRUG SAFETY

While preparing the previous section of my discussion I became more and more aware of the incredible shortage of accurate statistics. No doubt if I had had more time to study the literature a number of gaps would have been filled. Nevertheless, I suspect that even the most exhaustive search would reveal very few hard estimates of mortality in relation to drug therapy, and only a limited amount of information about the risks of disease.

In the long term I am convinced that it will be very difficult to obtain the information needed to balance risk and benefit until we have a much more comprehensive system for medical record linkage. It is sad that, although we probably have the finest health service in the world, we are still lamentably short of adequate statistics on which to base therapeutic decisions. Speaking tonight in the city of Oxford, I hardly need to remind you of the pioneer work by Donald Acheson who masterminded the Oxford Record Linkage scheme. His recent appointment as Chief Medical Officer brings the hope that the concept of **National Medical Record Linkage** might once again be revived. Donald was principally responsible for my move to Southampton to set up the Drug Surveillance Research Unit and it is a pleasure now to spend the remainder of this lecture describing some of the work we are doing and which he helped to make possible.

MEASURING THE RISKS AND BENEFITS

I have been privileged to have been closely involved in the development of both the monitoring schemes currently operating on a national scale. I was responsible for the CSM's "yellow card" scheme almost from the time it started in 1964 until 1980[9] and, subsequently, have set up a second system known as Prescription-Event Monitoring (PEM) at the University of Southampton[10,11]. The two schemes are complementary, the yellow cards enable "early warning" signals to be generated but do not usually allow incidence to be estimated, while PEM both generates signals and allows hypotheses to be tested.

Yellow Cards

Reply-paid "yellow cards" have been distributed to all doctors and dentists since 1964, and have provided a simple and effective means by which they can report suspected adverse drug reactions to the Committee on Safety of Medicines (CSM). At a recent meeting organized by the British Medical Association I was somewhat disturbed to hear the present Chairman of the CSM's Sub-Committee on Safety, Efficacy and Adverse Reactions say that the yellow card system is **not** an alerting system but, frankly, I would not have spent 16 years developing the system if I had believed this to have been true during that time. Certainly, yellow cards have identified a large number of potential safety problems. Only in exceptional circumstances, however, should the unvalidated reports be used as the sole reason for removing a drug from the market.

Yellow cards played a major role in the investigation of the safety of oral contraceptives. As early as 1964, doctors' reports suggested that thrombosis was occurring more frequently in women using the Pill. Moreover, they reported thrombosis in unusual sites such as the veins of the face or breast and diffuse multi-organ clotting. It was largely due to the efforts of the first Chairman of the Adverse Reaction Sub-Committee, the late Leslie Witts of this university, that studies were started by the Medical Research Council and the Royal College of General Practitioners which confirmed the results of the case-control study, set up by the Committee a year earlier, which had produced the first epidemiological evidence of probable association[12]. Subsequently, comparison of the yellow cards relating to certain brands of oral contraceptive showed a link with oestrogen dosage and this led, at the end of 1969, to the recommendation that only the smaller doses should be prescribed[13]. The Mini Pill, which followed, almost certainly eradicated this problem, and I believe that many tens of thousands of women throughout the world have reason to be grateful to the yellow card system.

Yellow cards are available from the moment the drug is first marketed and, provided doctors recognize or suspect adverse reactions and use the cards, they are still in my opinion the most effective method of drawing early attention to potential problems, especially if the adverse reactions are rare.

Prescription-event monitoring (PEM)

The concept of **event-monitoring** was first suggested by Professor David Finney as early as 1964, before the yellow card system was set up[14]. Recording adverse events, rather than merely suspicions that they might be drug-related, removes the need to give a medical opinion about the possible role of a drug in each adversity experienced by the patient.

Since the National Health Service started, the Prescription Pricing Authority has processed up to 300 million prescription forms each year, every one of which affords a unique opportunity to identify a doctor, a patient and one or more drug exposures. After the normal process of pricing has been completed, the prescriptions are stored for a few months and then destroyed.

Starting in 1978 I set about the task of convincing various official bodies, such as the DHSS and the BMA, that there should be no serious ethical or legal problems in using prescriptions in order to set up large groups of patients for subsequent study. In 1981 we commenced collecting copies of prescriptions in my Unit at Southampton. Questionnaires (green forms), which identify individual patients, are sent to GPs. Each form gives the following example of an event:

A broken leg is an EVENT. If more fractures were associated with this drug they could have been due to hypotension, CNS effects or metabolic bone changes.

Typically, we are investigating up to four drugs at any one time, we may identify up to 100,000 patients who have used any one of them. In order to reduce the burden of form-filling, we usually impose a limit of four patients (i.e. four green forms) per doctor per drug. We have had an enormous and very gratifying response, indeed, during the past 12 months we have received more than 100,000 green forms, exceeding the total input of yellow cards during the 16 years I was responsible for them. About three-quarters of all general practitioners in England are actively collaborating. Consistently, we have been able to study the pattern of events in groups of more than 10,000 patients. PEM can be used both to generate hypotheses and to test them and, as I hope to show you, the ability to compare events which occur while the patients are taking the drug and after they have stopped taking it also produces extremely valuable information about the background incidence of events[15].

As illustrations, I will now discuss how PEM reflects on three drugs: "Opren", "Zantac", and "Zomax".

"Opren" (benoxaprofen)

The ill-fated anti-arthritic drug, "Opren" was one of the first drugs subjected to PEM. We started to collect prescriptions in January 1981, and in January 1982 we launched a pilot study. Among approximately 6000 patients there were eight cases in which jaundice had been recorded as an event. Since a single case of jaundice always raises suspicion that a drug might be involved, I decided to follow up these eight cases before making any statement. At least five of them turned out to have nothing to do with the drug. Unfortunately, by the time these preliminary investigations were complete, "Opren" had become headline news and the drug was removed from the market in July 1982.

We included a further 18,000 patients in the study. Among them were 46 more cases. In the whole group of 24,000 patients (including those in the pilot study) there were 54 cases of jaundice or renal failure, 48 of whom were successfully followed up. Twenty-two patients had died, including three who had recovered from jaundice and died later from other causes. As can be seen in Table 3.6 the great majority turned out to have concurrent illnesses which could account for the jaundice or renal failure. These included cases of cancer of the pancreas, gall bladder or liver, gall stones, cirrhosis and infective hepatitis. At the end of the investigation, only a single case remained in which the drug could probably be blamed for jaundice and that was non-fatal. In addition there were 11 cases, including the six in which follow-up was still incomplete, where the drug might be regarded as a possible cause of jaundice or renal failure because alternative causes could not be completely ruled out.

The average period of treatment with "Opren" was about 6 months, and the period of follow-up after treatment had been discontinued averaged about 13 months. It is worth attempting to calculate the attributable and non-attributable risks of developing jaundice or renal failure in 700 per year, and the overall fatality rate, one in 1700 per year. If we assume that "Opren" was responsible in all 12 cases in which there was any possibility, however remote, that "Opren" might have been responsible, (including the six cases which have not been followed up), then the attributable case rate could be as large as about one in 1000 and the mortality rate about one in 2000. If instead we assume that "Opren" was responsible only in the single non-fatal case, which was probably due to "Opren", then that corresponds with an incidence of one attributable case in 12,000 patient-years of exposure to the drug, and no fatality.

Table 3.6 Follow-up of all cases of hepatic or renal failure occuring during or after treatment with benoxaprofen

Jaundice and/or renal failure	Cases identified in group of approximately 24,000 patients treated with benoxaprofen (deaths in parentheses)	
Probably due to benoxaprofen	1	
Possibly due to benoxaprofen	11*	(5)
Association unlikely	15	(6)
Unrelated	27	(11)
All cases	54	(22)

*Includes six cases rated "possible" by default, where no detailed information has been obtained.

It is important to note that even in this very large series it was impossible to arrive at a figure for the attributable mortality, and this suggests that fatal "Opren"-induced jaundice was in fact extremely rare. I do not believe that it was necessary to ban the drug simply because of the adverse publicity that had occurred. Many doctors commented during the course of our study on the very considerable benefit that their patients had experienced while taking "Opren". I believe that it was only necessary to react to the manufacturers report 12 months previously concerning slower metabolism by the elderly. A specific instruction about reducing the dose in elderly people had been circulated by the manufacturers and endorsed by the CSM a few weeks before the final removal of the drug.

"Zantac" (ranitidine)

My second example of Prescription-Event Monitoring in action is taken from a pilot study in more than 9000 patients who had been treated for peptic ulcer and dyspepsia with "Zantac" (ranitidine). The drug was effective in more than 70% of patients and the pattern of adverse events occurring after stopping the drug was not too different from that during treatment. There were, however, some intriguing differences when certain diagnoses were compared during the treatment and follow-up period. Everyday problems, such as rashes, anxiety or depression, respiratory infections or gynaecological disorders, occurred with roughly equal frequency during treatment and follow-up. Headache and dizziness were two to three times as common during treatment and these are recognized side-effects of the drug. Cholecystitis occurred about two and a half times more frequently than would have been expected. The cause of abdominal pain for which "Zantac" had been prescribed for some patients proved to have been gall stones. A more surprising finding was that orthopaedic surgery was three times more common during treatment. Patients on the waiting list for operations, such as total hip replacement, receive drugs to control the pain of their arthritis. These in turn cause dyspepsia for which "Zantac" had been prescribed! It was at this point that I began to feel that "real" patients were emerging from the mass of green forms we were accumulating.

"Zomax" (zomepirac)

My final example of PEM is drawn from a study of another anti-arthritic agent which was removed from the market after a small number of reports of anaphylactic shock. One patient who died was apparently related in some way to the owner of a television network, and publicity surrounding this single death led to its removal, first in the United States and, almost immediately afterwards, in this country.

The reported incidence of death from anaphylactic shock, worldwide, is about one in two million (placing this risk in level 7). No such deaths have been reported in patients taking "Zomax" in this country and in a study which we have conducted of nearly 10,000 patients, no deaths and only two non-fatal cases of anaphylaxis were recorded. Many patients had found the drug to be effective, including a group of some 400 patients with terminal cancer, many of whom suffered severely when the drug, which was unusually effective in controlling pain from secondary deposits in bone, was withdrawn. The pattern of adverse events was in no way remarkable in comparison with that for other drugs which we have studied, but we did make one exciting and potentially important discovery.

The removal of "Zomax" from the market, which was in no way related to the physical state of any of the patients, divided our study into two roughly equal parts. The 10,000 patients had been treated for about four months on average and followed up for a further four months after "Zomax" had been withdrawn. There were only minor differences in the pattern of most events during these periods. When, however, we came to compare cardiovascular mortality (Table 3.7), there appeared to be a striking **deficit** of deaths during the treatment period. Only one death from myocardial infarction was recorded during treatment but 12 were reported after it had been withdrawn from the market. If we included reports of fatal cerebrovascular accidents or pulmonary embolism, the ratio became one to 29. At first sight, this could represent a rebound effect due to withdrawal of the drug, but the number of deaths was consistent with the normal mortality from these causes when the age and duration of follow-up were taken into consideration. It seems much more likely that we are looking at a deficit of deaths during treatment rather than an excess after the end of treatment. We are currently investigating a larger number of deaths in which the cause was not reported on our green forms but which seem to have occurred mainly in the post-treatment period. This result makes biological sense because it is known that zomepirac affects certain enzymes and blood platelets in a way which would tend to diminish the risk of thrombosis[16]. Aspirin has been shown to exert some protective effect in myocardial infarction[17] and I was taught that people suffering from rheumatoid arthritis seem to be less prone to dying from heart attacks. This could be a result of the drugs they have used. This experience does suggest that PEM will almost certainly, from time to time, reveal important and unexpected benefits as well as possible dangers.

Table 3.7 Death from coronary disease, pulmonary embolism and stroke

Cardiovascular deaths	While on "Zomax"	After stopping "Zomax"
Coronary thrombosis	1	12
Pulmonary embolism	-	3
Stroke	-	14*
All deaths	1	29

*The proportion due to thrombosis or haemorrhage remains to be determined.

COMPARISON OF METHODS

In Figure 3.1 I have tried to show what risks might be detected by various methods of monitoring. Clinical trials and intensive monitoring schemes in hospitals, which are limited by the relatively small numbers of patients available for study, are likely only to measure risks in the first and second levels, in other words, those occurring in more than 1% of patients receiving a drug. Very occasionally, trials may be large enough to detect events occurring in the third risk level. PEM is limited only by the number of green forms that doctors might be persuaded to fill in. It has already taken us into level 4 and, if groups of more than 10,000 could be studied regularly, it could take us below this level, particularly if the need for doctors to transfer data from their notes to their green forms could be eliminated by automatic medical record linkage.

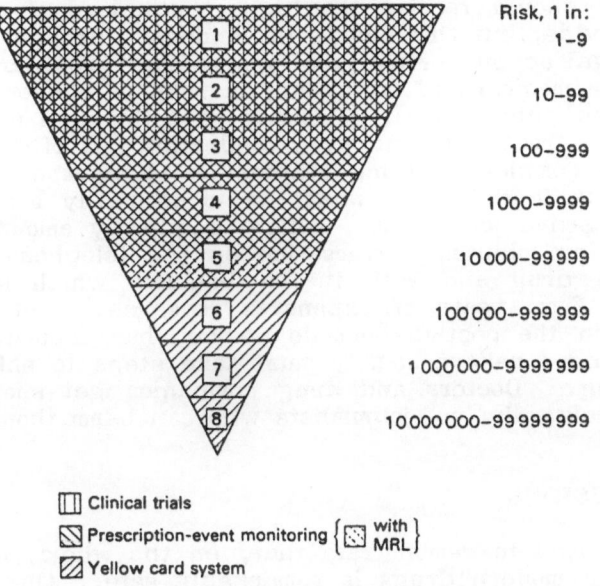

	Risk, 1 in:
1	1–9
2	10–99
3	100–999
4	1000–9999
5	10000–99999
6	100000–999999
7	1000000–9999999
8	10000000–99999999

▥ Clinical trials
▨ Prescription-event monitoring { ▧ with MRL }
▨ Yellow card system

Figure 3.1 Risk levels detectable by various methods of postmarketing surveillance

Only the yellow card system is potentially capable of detecting risks at all levels of incidence. There is no way that any nation could afford to set up comparative studies of millions of patients which would be required to detect risks at level 6 or below. Unfortunately, because of uncertainty about the completeness of reporting, yellow cards cannot estimate incidence. Nevertheless, they may allow us to make a reasonable guess at the probable risk level.

BARRIERS TO PROGRESS

There are many problems to be overcome, and I have selected four which I believe to be the most important. The first is **confidentiality**. In all my years of involvement in drug safety work I have never encountered a single case in which the transmission of confidential information from one doctor to another has harmed the patient. On the other hand I have encountered several situations in which delayed transmission of information has harmed many. Secondly, there are many **misconceptions** about safety and efficacy, largely induced by irresponsible reporting, which have created the myth that all drugs should be completely effective and totally safe.

Thirdly, there is the problem of **litigation**. I do not believe that the care of people who from time to time will inevitably be damaged by drugs, should be achieved by struggle through courts. Largely because of avarice in the United States, we are in danger of creating an elite of drug-damaged patients who feel they deserve astronomical sums of money in compensation. Whatever the cause of an injury, be it a drug or a banana skin, I believe that patients should receive the highest standard of care that society can provide, but this should be achieved through insurance rather than legal action. Finally, I believe that **premature publication**, in both the medical and lay press, is responsible for much suffering. It causes public alarm. It leads to withdrawal effects in patients who stop treatment, and even to deaths. It often makes it impossible to complete existing studies or to start new ones which will enable us to determine what the risks really are. Irresponsible "investigative journalism", which frequently amounts to little more than a few minutes conversation on the telephone, may destroy a valuable drug and with it the benefits which might have been derived from years of expensive research. Intervention by the media, in the post-thalidomide period, has caused more harm than good, and I believe society must take steps to enforce responsible reporting. Doctors and drug companies get sued for damage to individuals, why not journalists who can harm thousands?

CONCLUSIONS

I have tried to demonstrate that, on the whole, medical intervention with modern drugs is remarkably safe. Our main problem is not that risks outweigh benefits, it is that we cannot agree with each other about what risks are acceptable. Public opinion has swung much too far in the direction of excessive concern about rare side-effects, while common benefits are ignored. Perception of risks has been grossly distorted by horror stories. I once calculated that if **all** drug risks were eliminated, our average life expectancy might be increased by 37 minutes! This could be achieved by removing all therapeutically effective medicines and vaccines, but the cost in the end would be an average loss of life expectancy of perhaps 10 or 20 years.

We are dominated by our lack of good epidemiological data and by our inability to reach a consensus about which risks are important. Looking forward to the 21st century, I believe we should ensure that the next generation of prescribers will be equipped with the means of determining more precisely what the risks are. This can only be achieved through improved medical record linkage. Since Oxford has been a focal point for experiments in record linkage, I think that this is an appropriate place to end my lecture.

ACKNOWLEGEMENTS

I am deeply indebted to Dr John Urquhart, of Alza Corporation, Palo Alto, California, who inspired several of the ideas which I have incorporated in this lecture, and who let me read the then unpublished, "Keine Angst vor der Angst" (reference 8), which is a "must" for all students of risk and which should be compulsory reading for government officials, politicians, consumerists, and journalists. I would also like to thank Wolfson College and its President, Sir Henry Fisher, for inviting me to contribute to the 1984 series of lectures. These lectures, edited by Dr Michael Cooper, will be published by Oxford University Press later in the year and I am most grateful to the college and the publishers for permission to reproduce this lecture in full.

REFERENCES

1. Office of Population Censuses and Surveys (1983). Mortality Statistics, England and Wales 1981. (London: HMSO)
2. Urquhart, J and Heilmann, K Risk Watch. Understanding Risks in a Technological Society. (In press)
3. Inman, WHW (1981). Post-marketing surveillance. In Cavella, JF (ed.) Risk-Benefit Analysis in Drug Research. p.141-61 (Lancaster: MTP Press)
4. Rothschild (1978). The Listener. 30 November
5. Committee on Safety of Medicines (1982)
6. Second Benoxaprofen Symposium. 15th International Rheumatology Congress. Paris, June 1981. Europ J Rheumatol Inflamm (1982) 5(2) 49-282
7. Inman, WHW (1977). Study of fatal bone marrow depression with special reference to phenylbutazone and oxyphen-butazone. Br Med J, 1, 1500-5
8. Heilmann, K and Urquhart, J (1983). Keine Angst vor der Angst. (Munich: Kindler Verlag)
9. Inman, WHW (1980). (ed.). Monitoring for Drug Safety. (Lancaster: MTP Press)
10. Inman, WHW (1981). Post-marketing surveillance of adverse drug reactions in general practice. I: Search for new methods. Br Med J, 282, 1131-2
11. Inman, WHW (1981). Post-marketing surveillance of adverse drug reactions in general practice. II: Prescription-event monitoring at the University of Southampton. Br Med J, 282, 1216-7
12. Inman, WHW and Vessey, MP (1968). Investigation of deaths from pulmonary, coronary and cerebral thrombosis and embolism in women of child-bearing age. Br Med J, 2, 193-9
13. Inman, WHW, Vessey, MP, Westerholm, B and Engelund, A (1970). Thromboembolic disease and the steroidal content of oral contraceptives. A report to the Committee on Safety of Medicines. Br Med J, 2, 203-9
14. Finney, DJ (1965). The design and logic of a monitor of drug use. J Chron Dis, 18, 77-98
15. Drug Surveillance Research Unit (1983). PEM News, No. 1, (Southampton: Hamble Valley Press)
16. Hook, BG, Rumson, JL, Jolly SR, Bailie, MB and Lucchesi, BR (1983). Effect of Zomepirac on experimental coronary ar-

tery thrombosis and ischaemic myocardial injury in the conscious dog. J Cardiovasc Pharmacol, 5, 302-8

17.   Lewis, HD et al. (1983).   Protective effects of aspirin against acute myocardial infarction and death in men with unstable angina. N Engl J Med, 309(7), 396-403

4

The Use of Human Biological Measurements for Safety Evaluation in the Chemical Industry

W. HOWE, M. D. STONARD AND B. H. WOOLLEN

INTRODUCTION

Although man has been exposed to naturally occurring poisons since the beginning of his existence, it is only in the past 80 years that there has been a dramatic increase in the number of synthetic chemicals, a few of which have subsequently been shown to cause health problems following human exposure. However, health in this country is better than in past times and the expectation of life in this chemical age is longer than ever before[1]. There is no evidence of mass harm to the population from new substances[2,3]. In the chemical industry, past history has shown that health effects have usually resulted from specific exposures; for example: bladder cancer from exposure to aromatic amines, fibrotic lung disease from exposure to silica dust, mesothelioma from asbestos, occupational asthma from exposure to platinum salts and more recently angiosarcoma of the liver from exposure to vinyl chloride monomer. As well as in the industrial situation, man is exposed to chemicals in pharmaceutical preparations, domestic products, food additives, pesticide residues and from accidental contamination of the environment.

Risks to health following chemical exposure have been recognized either by the astute physician relating clinical cases to particular substances, from mortality or morbidity statistics or from prospective or retrospective epidemiological studies[4]. In the chemical industry we define a **hazard** as the potential for a substance to produce adverse health effects, and **risk** as the probability of a substance causing harm to an individual in the circumstances in which he is being exposed. The problem in relying on the assessment of health risks, as described above, is that harmful exposures have to occur before a health effect is demonstrated, and if chronic effects are produced it may take many years before the causative agent is identified.

To overcome this delay, model test systems, using either animal bioassays or in vitro methods, have been developed to try and predict hazard to man before harmful exposure occurs. In

63

animal studies, doses of the chemical are normally administered either orally, by skin application or by inhalation, and any biological effects observed. By using a range of doses a "no-effect level" can be determined and a dose/response relationship established. An assessment of the hazard to humans exposed to the chemical can be derived from these data, categorizing substances into different general classes, e.g. toxic, corrosive, carcinogenic. Standards for acceptable human exposure can be derived by determining the highest dose which causes no effect in animals, and either introducing safety margins arbitrarily or by using mathematical models. For example, in the chemical industry a major route of exposure to toxic substances is by the inhalation of gases, dusts or vapours and traditionally "safe" working conditions have been related to standards for atmospheric contamination through monitoring the environment to demonstrate compliance with these standards[5,6]. However, atmospheric monitoring has several limitations. It only monitors the overall airborne potential for exposure and not the actual total exposure of individuals; therefore it is unsuitable for substances absorbed through the skin.

When using animal data to set these standards it is assumed that any observed biological effect is related to the dose administered. Initially it must be assumed that the absorption, metabolism, excretion and the biological effect in man are qualitatively similar to those occurring in animals. However, quantitative extrapolation to a situation of actual exposure is often difficult because of unrealistically high doses used in animal toxicity studies, inappropriate routes of administration, poor or unknown bioavailability, or differences in routes of biotransformation. Furthermore differences in response are often found between animal species and in the absence of any information to the contrary the most sensitive species must be used as a model for man, even though this may in fact be totally inappropriate. Such factors may result in the hazard assessment being invalid, safe exposure standards being set at an inappropriate level or a decision being taken that the chemical should not be manufactured or used.

Whilst the use of animal bioassays is adequate for assessing risk prior to human exposure to most chemicals, there still remains, for some chemicals, a need for post-exposure surveillance of humans in order to identify whether any adverse health effects are occurring[7]. Ideally a more systematic and rapid approach for estimating risk to humans should be developed rather than waiting for the findings from human epidemiological studies. The measurement of pharmacokinetic parameters (absorption, distribution, biotransformation and elimination) in both animals and humans is clearly established as part of the safety evaluation process in the pharmaceutical industry where novel substances are intended for use in man. A similar approach can be applied to the study of industrial chemicals in man. The pharmacokinetic profile may then be used to develop a rational strategy for monitoring the levels of chemical which are absorbed following incidental exposure in the workplace.

Although this process will allow concentrations measured in animal studies to be extrapolated more accurately to man, there is also a need in human post-exposure surveillance to relate concentrations of chemicals to biological effects. Chemicals may produce specific effects, for instance, by direct interaction with an enzyme in a metabolic pathway which results in an abnormally high production of an endogenous substance that can be measured conveniently. However, it is more common to employ a battery of tests which reflect structural and functional abnormalities in the target organ, e.g. serum analysis for hepatic dysfunction and urine analysis for renal dysfunction. In future it will be important to identify a wider range of parameters which are affected by specific chemicals and devise methods to measure these parameters at a stage when they are both subclinical and reversible[8]. A knowledge of the concentrations of chemicals producing these effects will permit dose-effect/response relationships to be derived and biological standards to be established, so that strategies for monitoring procedures can be used to demonstrate safe working practices.

At their Central Toxicology Laboratory, ICI has recognized the importance of the above concepts as part of the safety evaluation of chemicals, and has established a research team to gather more data on exposure, absorption, biotransformation and elimination of chemicals in man. These data can then be related to similar parameters in laboratory animal studies and to occupationally related measurements of dysfunction in order to make more quantitative risk assessments as a basis for biological monitoring procedures.

The future approach to safety evaluation will now be considered under the broad areas of exposure, absorption, biological monitoring and biological effects.

EXPOSURE

Atmospheric monitoring provides a satisfactory way of assessing the potential exposure of many chemicals, particularly those which are present in the workplace as vapours and dusts. It is, however, an inappropriate way of estimating exposure to chemicals which are mainly absorbed by routes other than inhalation (e.g. dermal).

Some attempts have been made to assess potential dermal exposure to industrial chemicals but far more extensive work has been carried out on estimating exposure to pesticides[9]. Methods used involve fixed pads or disposable paper suits which are worn by operators during exposure, and which are subsequently analysed for their content of the active ingredient. Using such techniques it is possible to pinpoint which parts of the body receive the highest degree of exposure[10]. For a given method of application and certain types of formulation a data base is being established which can be used to estimate the dermal exposure to pesticides without the necessity to carry out repetitive field trials. Techniques have also been developed to allow the use of in vitro permeability measurements with intact human skin to predict the rate of absorption of pesticides in vivo[11,12]. By applying the measured rate of penetration from such studies to the surface area of the exposed body parts and adjusting for the duration of exposure a potential absorbed dose can be predicted. Industrial chemicals differ from pesticides in that dermal exposure is likely to be incidental and the pattern of work less predictable. However, some of the methods developed for pesticides are likely to be of value in assessing exposure of individual workers to industrial chemicals, and the measurement of skin permeability should play a role in assessing potential dermal uptake.

ABSORPTION

The proportion of an available chemical that is absorbed by the body can vary substantially depending on the route of administration. Therefore an assessment of total dermal exposure may greatly overestimate the amount actually absorbed. Hence more accurate ways are needed for assessing the amount of a chemical absorbed in exposed persons, in order to improve the assessment of the probability that a toxic response will occur.

The dose of a chemical delivered to the specific target tissue (animal or human) is the factor most closely related to a toxic response[7,13]. Although this tissue dose can be determined in animal studies it is difficult to estimate in humans because of the limitations of available sampling techniques. The application of pharmacokinetic analysis is one method of overcoming this problem as both the concentration of active substance in body fluids and also the quantity absorbed over a given time period can be estimated[14].

It has been shown that the blood concentrations of unchanged drugs reflect in most instances the dose which reaches the target site, and this principle can be applied to industrial chemicals to give a better estimate of tissue dose than can be achieved by direct measurements of potential uptake[15]. However difficulties sometimes arise in interpreting the results of such measurements in an absence of a full understanding of the metabolism of a chemical and its relationship to the mechanism of toxicity. Nevertheless by comparing human pharmacokinetic data with those derived from animal studies it is possible to carry out an improved semi-quantitative safety evaluation[14]. Data from human studies involving small doses of chemicals will allow bioavailability, volume of distribution, metabolic profile and route and rate of elimination to be compared with animal kinetic experiments. If there are similarities, then it is possible to carry out a risk assessment by making comparisons of both peak blood levels and estimates of absorption. The latter can be estimated from the area under the curve (AUC) for a blood concentration v. time plot, or from measurements of compound or metabolites in urine. Data generated from blood and urine measurements in exposed workers can then be compared with similar data from animals exposed at a no-effect dose level. The magnitude of the safety margins derived from these comparisons can be used to assist in establishing safe working practices.

Recent studies have been carried out by the laboratory on an exploratory assessment of the degree of absorption of dinitrotoluene (DNT) by exposed workers[16]. A major metabolite, 2,4-dinitrobenzoic acid (2,4-DNBA), was present in urine samples from exposed workers but the concentrations did not accumulate during a working week and returned to low or non-detectable levels at the beginning of the next working week. Analysis of consecutive samples showed that the highest levels of 2,4-DNBA were found in urine collected at the end of shift.

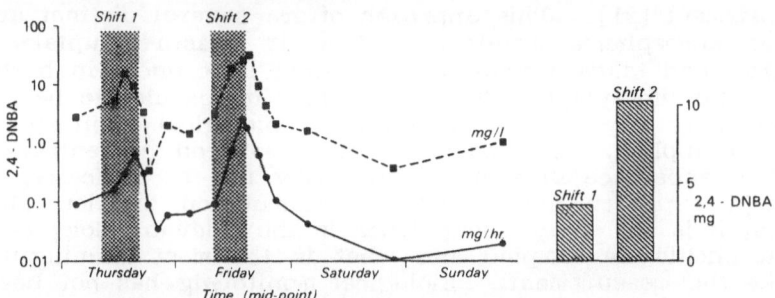

Figure 4.1 Semi-logarithmic plot 2,4-DNBA excreted by a process worker over a 4-day period. In the graphs the working periods are shaded. The bar charts indicate the amounts of 2,4-DNBA excreted in urine during the 24-hour periods including the two workshifts

Although the results demonstrate that DNT absorption is occurring, it is not possible to estimate the total absorbed dose since the proportion of DNT converted to 2,4-DNBA is not known. A controlled human dosing study would be needed to obtain this information.

Prior to this survey it was believed that adherence to prescribed atmospheric limits for DNT would prevent significant absorption; however, the study indicates that skin is the major route of uptake, and appropriate action has been taken to reduce exposure.

Studies involving comparative pharmacokinetics have been carried out for pesticides and for some industrial chemicals[15]. Similarities in pharmacokinetics between man and experimental animals were used[17] to establish an adequate safety margin for spray operators exposed to 2,4,5-T. Human studies have also been carried out involving the administration of pesticides by the dermal route in cases where this was believed to be a likely route of uptake[18,19]. For the herbicide picloram only 0.2% of the applied dose was absorbed by the dermal route, whereas most of the dose was absorbed after oral administration[18]. Similar studies are needed for selected industrial chemicals to bridge the gap between incomplete measurements of human incidental exposure and the results of animal dosing studies. The use of comparative pharmacokinetics can be time-consuming and the interpretation of the results may be difficult. Hence in the first instance they will only be used to answer specific problems. However, this approach offers the best means of satisfying the needs of industry and society for more accurate assessment of safety, in the limited number of cases where existing methods are inadequate[20].

BIOLOGICAL MONITORING

The opportunity to establish biological monitoring procedures follows naturally from the assessment of comparative pharmacokinetics. Biological monitoring can be defined as "a regular measuring activity where selected validated indicators of uptake of toxic substances are determined in order to prevent health impairment"[21]. This approach offers several distinct advantages over atmospheric monitoring since it measures uptake from all routes and takes account of individual differences in both metabolism and lifestyle[7,22-25]. However, it has also to be recognized that there are several limitations to biological monitoring as currently applied. For example, the measured concentration of the active substance in a body fluid may not be indicative solely of recent exposure due to either accumulation or slow elimination. Also, it is not always clear which is the relevant biological material that should be sampled and what is the most meaningful time to make the measurement. Biological monitoring has not been widely adopted by the chemical industry and this is reflected in the small number of substances for which monitoring strategies are established.

Despite these difficulties, biological monitoring will be used increasingly to assess actual worker absorption of chemicals where it has been identified that a hazard of particular concern exists. This applies both to established products whose risk may need to be re-evaluated on the basis of new data from animal toxicity studies and also to new products.

Biological threshold limit values (BTLV) were introduced initially for existing substances such as lead and mercury. In 1984 the American Conference of Governmental Industrial Hygienists published some proposed BTLVs for industrial chemicals such as trichloroethylene, styrene and carbon monoxide[26]. It seems inevitable that the introduction of biological threshold values will grow rapidly during the next few years. It must be emphasized that these thresholds have been, and can only be, defined if there is a satisfactory animal and human data base for the relationship between absorbed dose and biological effect for these chemicals. Key chemicals which need to be investigated in terms of absorption and effect in man will be identified on the basis of toxicity in animals, annual volume of production, the number of people exposed during production and usage, and structure/activity relationships.

As biological monitoring gains more widespread acceptance it will be used as part of an overall programme of worker health protection. This process will be facilitated where possible by the development of rapid, simple and specific tests for routine use. These tests will be applied to blood and urine but also increasingly to other biological samples which can be obtained by non-invasive sampling. For example, the use of saliva as a non-invasive medium for evaluating absorbed doses of chemicals merits further attention, especially as saliva may be provided more conveniently than blood in the workplace. Specific breathalysers for industrial chemicals (either colour-indicating or based on a physical or biological property of the component of interest) will be introduced to control exposure to certain chemicals where breath is demonstrated to be a reliable way of assessing absorption. Using silicon wafer etching technology it is now possible to make a gas chromatograph the size of a matchbox[27], and such separation devices could be incorporated in portable breath analysis systems. Miniature portable mass spectrometers, which provide a combination of high sensitivity with extremely high specificity, have also been shown to have a tremendous potential for breath monitoring[28].

An area of biological monitoring which will undoubtedly assume increasing importance in the future is the measurement of stable covalent adducts formed by the interaction of electrophilic substances with proteins and DNA. The concept of measuring the concentration of protein adducts between electrophiles and certain amino acids in haemoglobin as an index of integrated exposure to chemicals is practicable because haemoglobin in circulating erythrocytes[29] has a biological half-life of approximately 120 days.

This strategy has been used already to demonstrate a correlation between occupational exposure and alkylation of histidine for ethylene and propylene oxides[30,31]. The potential interaction of electrophiles with nucleophilic centres on all four DNA bases poses a daunting analytical challenge. DNA adduct formation offers a promising approach to estimating the actual amount of a toxic substance which is absorbed and reaches cellular macromolecules, but so far it has only been applied to the measurement of degradation products of modified DNA in rat urine[32].

The application of biological monitoring to covalent adducts is limited, at present, by its relative insensitivity and time-consuming sample preparation procedures prior to the sophisticated GC-MS instrumentation required for the final analysis. However, immunological techniques are being developed which offer several advantages: with the advent of hybridoma technology, monoclonal antibodies directed against electrophile-hybridoma DNA adducts offer a rapid, specific and highly sensitive approach to estimating absorbed doses of chemicals in chronic low-level exposure situations.

Although measurements of parent compound and active metabolite levels will continue to be made in the more accessible body fluids such as blood and urine, for certain substances, e.g. toxic metals, the inherent limitations of such analyses without the corresponding tissue analyses have been recognized and attention has now focused on the potential use of sophisticated non-invasive methods of analysis in target organs. For example, significant progress has been made in measuring the concentrations of cadmium in liver and kidneys of exposed workers using a portable neutron activation analysis system[33-35]. This same principle is being applied to the determination of mercury in tissue but an order of magnitude improvement in sensitivity is required before the method can be applied more widely[36]. An alternative technique, X-ray fluorescence, has already been investigated for various elements in organs either on the surface or just under the skin. It is being successfully applied to the measurement of mercury in superficial tissues of the head[37], but appears less suitable at present for monitoring mercury in an organ such as the kidney which lies some 3-5 cm below the skin surface[36]. Further development of these techniques will take place to lower the detection limits.

BIOLOGICAL EFFECTS

Early markers of cellular damage or organ dysfunction constitute an important and expanding area of human biological measurements. The primary objective remains the identification of specific biological events which give a warning of potential for more serious health effects in both the general population and specific occupational groups. It is envisaged that future emphasis will be placed upon the detection of subclinical effects in several organ systems. Although organs such as the liver, kidney and lung will continue to receive attention, it is apparent that other target organs such as the reproductive tract and the nervous system, and screening for genotoxic events, will attract further attention as new methods are developed.

One of the major problems in these areas is the lack of established "normal values" for many of these parameters. A need exists to define normality and to define the health significance of deviations from these values. The need for "normal values" is well illustrated from our own experience. In 1980 ICI established a mobile lung function unit to conduct epidemiological surveys of lung function of company employees. This facility, which is capable of measuring variables of ventilation, distribution and gas exchange, has been used recently in an extensive lung function study to derive normal values for employees in chemical manufacture. The results of this survey (Tams, personal communication) indicate considerable differences from similar measurements made in the USA[38,39]. Furthermore, differences exist in predictive values derived from cross-sectional studies compared with longitudinal studies. This survey serves to underline the importance of establishing normal values for all biological parameters which are to be evaluated subsequently in exposed populations. These new data now form a firm basis for further studies of lung function within the British chemical industry.

Chromosomal analysis of peripheral human lymphocytes is the most widely used approach for monitoring human populations exposed to genotoxic chemicals. Although the observation of chromosome changes in these cells is difficult to relate to future changes in phenotypic expression, e.g. cancer, this technique nevertheless continues to provide evidence for the presence of genetically active material in the individual. A detailed analysis of over 100 human surveillance cytogenetic studies[40], has highlighted several shortcomings which require immediate attention. In particular, measurements and reporting techniques associated with the assay system require standardization in order to obtain more reliable and less variable baseline data. An alternative genetic end-point is the induction of sister chromatid exchange (SCE). This approach still requires further development and validation but the potential application of SCE in genetic monitoring can be gauged from a study of vinyl chloride workers in which SCEs returned to normal as improvements in industrial hygiene measures were implemented[41]. However, the uncertainty about the phenotypic significance of elevated SCEs and the presence of confounding factors such as smoking and lifestyle may prove to be obstacles to wider acceptance of the technique[42]. As the major industrial genotoxic chemicals have been identified and either removed from use or exposures markedly reduced, the ability to detect untoward genotoxic effects in humans becomes technically more difficult. The cytogenetic techniques employed will need to be sufficiently sensitive to detect changes related to exposure which are greater than individual variability. The most effective way forward appears to involve the simultaneous evaluation of more than one cytogenetic end-point in groups of workers considered at risk in the occupational environment or individuals with accidental exposure to known mutagens/carcinogens. In the longer term it seems likely that molecular biology will provide parameters which link chemical effects on DNA more specifically with aspects of the mechanism of cancer induction.

There has been growing concern, some of which appears unfounded, that a number of chemicals may induce infertility by damage to the reproductive tract, especially in males[43], e.g. 1,2-dibromo-3-chloropropane. Within the complex process of reproduction several functional end-points can be recognized, but the quality and quantity of information which may be gathered in humans is governed in large part by the degree of access to suitable biological materials, e.g. semen. Although the induction of morphologically abnormal sperm provides tentative evidence of an adverse effect, screening procedures that assess critical aspects of sperm function will be invaluable for correlating structure-function relationships. Future studies of testicular function will need to include not only a detailed occupational and reproductive history from both partners, but also relevant blood hormone levels (gonadotrophins and testosterone) together with information on sperm numbers, morphological appearance, motility and fertilizing capacity. Forward progressive motility is probably the single most important parameter of sperm for assessing fertility[44]. Studies of female reproductive function will depend upon a comprehensive history of the menstrual cycle and any disorders, hormonal status (oestrogen and progesterone levels in blood and urine) and, where appropriate, studies of cyclical changes in cervical mucus and endometrial morphology.

Considerable effort should be directed towards the identification of biological markers which are early indicators of chemically induced reproductive dysfunction. Possible markers which may be useful include certain organ-specific enzymes and proteins which may be released into body fluids when damage occurs. The foundations for such an approach have already been laid by the two-dimensional mapping of proteins in human seminal fluid[45] and human testis[46]. Also, the application of monoclonal antibodies directed against "immature" or abnormal sperm in human semen, and the identification of antigenic determinants involved in fertilization, may provide us with an alternative approach to the early detection of chemically induced reproductive dysfunction.

Although the potential for chemicals to produce reproductive toxicity and genotoxicity are emotive and contemporary issues, there is also an increased public awareness of the problems of gradual loss of cognitive functions that may occur in individuals occupationally exposed to various chemicals.

Several chemicals of diverse structure may produce subtle effects long before any clinical signs are manifest, and the early detection of these effects of the nervous system and on the psychological status will place additional demands on occupational health practice. Because nervous system syndromes may only develop slowly via a progressive loss of compensatory mechanisms in the nervous system, and considerable inter-individual variability in response exists, the detection of these subclinical effects is dependent upon the nature and sensitivity of the laboratory and clinical examinations employed. However, this approach highlights the core problem of neuropsychological research - that the more sensitive the method, the less specific the results.

Several Scandinavian studies have purported to show that chronic exposure to several solvent mixtures may contribute to an organic brain syndrome characterized by impairment of memory and co-ordination and some deterioration of personality[47]. The scientific basis upon which these claims have been made has been challenged in a recent review of the available literature[48]. These authors have critically evaluated the current techniques used in the investigation of personality, intelligence and memory, and have concluded that although the techniques are of value in the clinical examination of individual patients, they are unsuitable at present in epidemiological studies. The controversy surrounding the alleged existence of this organic brain syndrome is unlikely to be resolved until an exhaustive and critical evaluation of current methods is undertaken. The development and application of neurobehavioural methods in occupational health has been discussed at a recent international symposium[49]. Several conclusions and pointers for the future can be drawn from the meeting. One of the main problems in many electrophysiological studies remains the definition of normal values, and of the lower limits in healthy persons. Artifacts arising from both technical procedures and experimental design appear commonplace. In future studies it is important that rigorous standardization of methods is undertaken between competent laboratories in order to reduce inherent variability. Also, in order to compare the relative merits of different neurological function (CNS, PNS and behavioural/cognitive) should be specified. Although some techniques appear robust and offer valuable information in epidemiological studies, others appear inadequate for a variety of reasons - lack of sensitivity and specificity, irreproducibility, cumbersome to perform. It has also to be recognized that behavioural alterations may be produced by other factors, and that interpretation of future studies will need to take account of general aspects of lifestyle including ageing, shiftwork, excessive alcohol intake, psychoactive drugs, problems in interhuman relationships, etc.

Several new techniques have made in vivo imaging of whole organs a reality. The introduction of computerized tomography (CT), which consists of scanning narrow slices of tissue by a beam of X-rays, opens up the potential for assessing early stages of organ damage[50].   However, it is envisaged that CT and other sophisticated techniques such as nuclear magnetic resonance[51] and regional cerebral blood flow measurements[52] with xenon-133 will find increasing application for small groups of workers who are considered to be at risk from specific chemicals.   These techniques will not be suitable for screening large populations.

Considerable interest has been aroused by the recent introduction of an elegant two-dimensional technique for separating complex mixtures of proteins in biological systems[53].   The technique is being exploited in several directions.   The cataloguing of different proteins in various cell types brings nearer the ultimate goal of a total human protein map.   However, on a more realistic level the technique has the potential to identify subtle changes in protein composition, and as such appears admirably suited to the detection of early-effect markers of disease processes.   The identification of a novel protein change which relates to selective damage to an organ, will lead to the isolation and characterization of the protein, and the raising of an antibody for its quantitative measurement.   The directions in which the technique can be utilized appear numerous.   For instance it offers the possibility of detecting point mutations over larger regions of coding DNA than are presently monitored by any alternative method[54].   The technique is currently being employed to screen serum samples from individuals participating in the Janus project[55].   This project was initiated by the Norwegian Cancer Society in 1973 and has involved the collection and storage of blood samples at regular intervals from some 60,000 individuals.   For those individuals in the project who subsequently develop cancer, it is possible to look for changes in protein composition which may serve as early markers of an impending carcinogenic event.   If this project proves successful,   then this concept may find eventual application to screening employees in the chemical industry.

There are several well-established examples of genetic predisposition to diseases caused by drugs and chemicals[56].   The detection of individuals who may be genetically predisposed to disease, will be made possible by the application of DNA probes. These probes - consisting of a portion of DNA which can be tagged, e.g. with a radiolabel - are being used to identify similar portions of DNA in other test systems by hybridization techniques. It is now possible to extract DNA from peripheral lymphocytes and to use hybridization techniques to probe the DNA characteristics of these cells.   If relatively simple assays which use DNA probes can be devised to identify individuals at greater risk, then it will become necessary to consider the social and ethical implications of introducing such tests in pre-employment screening programmes. More recently a number of in vitro test systems for assessing hazard have been developed.   Tests for mutational effects are well established where either bacterial or mammalian cell cultures are tested with chemicals and semi-quantitative dose/response relationships derived.   Other short-term in vitro cell test systems are now being developed in our laboratory to identify the effect of chemicals on liver, testicular, and skin cell cultures as well as tests to demonstrate immunological effects.   The results of these tests and other developments will increasingly play a part in the safety evaluation of chemicals (Table 4.1).

Table 4.1 Future development of safety evaluation

Requirement	Existing approach	Future enhancements
Hazard assessment	Animal testing	Preliminary toxicity screen(in vitro)
	Clinical effects	
Risk assessment	Adequate safety margins	Comparative pharmacokinetics
	"No": Abandon "Yes": Establish exposure standard	Estimates of dermal exposure Identify sub-clinical effect Markers and define normal values
Risk management	Atmospheric monitoring	Biological monitoring
	Clinical health surveillance	Sub-clinical health surveillance
	Epidemiology	

The interpretation of biological measurements will become more exact as more data accumulate. Some conclusions will only be drawn by the study of large numbers of results using epidemiological techniques. It is important that effective use is made of the new data-handling technology to make it easier to carry out such summaries. A need will always exist to draw together information on the chemicals to which man has been exposed, the extent of the exposure, the degree of absorption and any health effects. The use of computerized record systems, allowing interactive searching, is an important development in this area. This is especially important in measuring health effects when baseline measurements are required before men begin work in a particular chemical environment.

CONCLUSIONS

Managers in the chemical industry have to establish a reasonable balance between acceptable risk to the workforce, benefit to society and profitability when deciding on viable chemical processes. In some cases, if the degree of worker exposure to a chemical cannot be reduced to acceptable levels, decisions may be necessary to close down certain processes or seek alternative synthetic routes. As in the past, hazardous and uneconomic processes will be replaced by new areas of business. The potential hazards from such new industries, e.g. biotechnology, electronics, have not yet been fully defined and continued vigilance is needed to identify any problems which may arise[57]. The application of modern engineering standards to new manufacturing processes, and an increased use of automation and robotics, should gradually reduce worker exposure to all chemicals in the future.

Human volunteer dosing studies with selected chemicals will be necessary if safety evaluation is to be improved. Such studies should be based on good scientific principles and ethical considerations, taking adequate account of the available animal toxicity data. Under these circumstances the risk to health must always be small compared to the scientific benefit which accrues in occupational health assessment.

In conclusion, we advocate the need for further studies on selected chemicals both in human volunteers and occupationally exposed individuals, on the basis that only tentative reliance may be placed on predictions of human response which depend exclusively on animal toxicology studies.

Further studies should be designed to provide comparative kinetic data, and to define normal values for biochemical, physiological and psychological parameters. The measurement of the absorption of a chemical and the demonstration of the resultant response in humans will remain the ultimate assessment of actual risk in exposed individuals.

REFERENCES

1. McLean, AEM (1981). Quantification of biological risk. Proc R Soc Lond, A376, 51-64
2. Doll, R (1979). The pattern of disease in the post-infection area: national trends, Proc R Soc Lond, B205, 47-61
3. DHSS (1978). Inequalities in Health. Department of Health and Social Security publication, p.75
4. McDonald, JC and Harrington, JM (1981). Early detection of occupational hazards. J Soc Occup Med, 31, 93-8
5. Occupational Exposure Limits. EH40 Health and Safety Executive (1984). (London: HMSO)
6. Monitoring Strategies for Toxic Substances. EH42 Health and Safety Executive (1984). (London: HMSO)
7. Lauwerys, RR (1983). Industrial Chemical Exposure: Guidelines for Biological Monitoring. (Biomedical Publications)
8. Taylor, W (1979). Man and his job. Br Med J, 2, 1066-7
9. Einert, C, Adams, W, Crothers, R, Moore, H and Ottoboni, F (1963). Exposure to mixtures of nitro-glycerin and ethylene glycol dinitrate. Am Ind Hyg Assoc J, 24, 435-47
10. World Health Organization (1982). Field Surveys of Exposure to Pesticides. Standard Protocol VBC/82.1
11. Dugard, PH (1983). Skin permeability theory in relation to measurements of percutaneous absorption in toxicology. In

Marzulli, FN and Maibach, HI (eds) Dermatotoxicology, 2nd Edn. pp. 91-116. (London: Hemisphere)

12. Bronaugh, RL and Maibach, HI (1983). In vitro percutaneous absorption. In Marzulli, FN and Maibach, HI (eds) Dermatotoxicology, 2nd Edn. (London: Hemisphere)

13. Starr, TB and Gibson, JE (1984). The importance of delivered dose in quantitative risk estimation: Formaldehyde. Toxicologist, 4, 30

14. Case, DE (1981). The state of the art: a commentary on the current practice of metabolism and pharmaco-kinetic studies in the pharmaceuticals industry. Xenobiotica, 11, 803-14

15. Watanabe, PG, Ramsey, JC and Gehring, PJ (1980). Pharmacokinetics and metabolism of industrial chemicals. In Bridges, JW and Chasseaud, LF (eds) Progress in Drug Metabolism, 5, 311-43. (Chichester: Wiley Interscience)

16. Woollen, BH, Hall, MG, Craig, R and Steel, GT (1986). Dinitrotoluene: an assessment of occupational absorption during the manufacture of blasting explosives. Int Arch Occup Environ Hlth (In press)

17. Leng, ML, Ramsey, JC, Braun, WH and Levy, TL (1982). Review of studies with 2,4,5-trichloro-phenoxyacetic acid in humans including applicators under field conditions. In Plimmer, JR (ed.) ACS Symposium Series. Pesticide Residues and Exposure, 182, 132-56. (Washington: American Chemical Society)

18. Nolan, RJ, Freshour, NL, Kaste, PE and Saunders, JH (1984). Pharmacokinetics of picloram in human volunteers. Tox Appl Pharmacol, 76, 264-9

19. Kolmodin-Hedman, B, Hoglund, S, Swensson, A and Akerblom, M (1983). Studies on phenoxy acid herbicides II. Oral and dermal uptake and elimination in urine of MCPA in humans. Arch Toxicol, 54, 267-73

20. Waldron, HA (1985). Which way ahead? Br J Industr Med, 42, 1-2

21. Tola, S and Hernberg, S (1981). Strategies for biological monitoring. In McDonald, JC (ed.) Recent Advances in Occupational Health. pp. 185-97. (London: Churchill Livingstone)

22. Zielhuis, RL (1978). Biological monitoring. Scand J Work Environ Hlth, 4 1-18

23. Berlin, A, Yodaiken, Re and Henman, BA (1984). Assessment of Toxic Agents at the Workplace: Roles of Ambient and Biological Monitoring (Amsterdam: Martinus Nijhoff, for the Commission of the European Communities)

24. Baselt, RC (1980). Biological Monitoring Methods for Industrial Chemicals. (Biomedical Publications)

25. Aitio, A, Riihimaki, V and Vainio, H (eds) (1984). Biological Monitoring and Surveillance of Workers Exposed to Chemicals. (London: Hemisphere)

26. American Conference of Governmental Industrial Hygienists (1984-1985). TLVs: Threshold Limit Values for Chemical Substances and Physical Agents in the Work Environment and Biological Exposure Indices with Intended Changes for 1984-85, second printing

27.   Angell, JB, Terry, SC and Barth, PW (1983).   Silicon
      microchip devices. Sci Am, April, pp. 36-45
28.   Wilson, HK and Ottley, TW (1981).   The use of a transport-
      able mass spectrometer in the direct measurement of industrial
      solvents in breath. Biomed Mass Spectrom, 8, 606-10
29.   Ehrenberg, L (1979).   Risk assessment of ethylene oxide and
      other compounds. In McElheny, VK and Abrahamson, S (eds)
      Banbury Report I: Assessing Chemical Mutagens: The Risk to
      Humans. pp. 157-90. (New York: Cold Spring Harbor
      Laboratory)
30.   Calleman, CJ, Ehrenberg, L and Jansson, B (1978).   Monitor-
      ing and risk assessment by means of alkyl groups in
      haemoglobin in persons occupationally exposed to ethylene
      oxide. J Environ Pathol Toxicol, 2, 427-42
31.   Osterman-Golkar, S, Bailey, E, Farmer, P, Gorf, SM and
      Lamb, JH (1984).   Monitoring exposure to propylene oxide
      through the determination of haemoglobin alkylation. Scand J
      Work Environ Hlth, 10, 99-102
32.   Shuker, DE, Bailey, E, Gorf, S, Lamb, J and Farmer, PB
      (1984).   Determination of N-7-[$^{2}H_3$]methyl guanine in rat
      urine by gas chromatography-mass spectrometry following ad-
      ministration of trideuteromethylating agents or precursors.
      Anal Biochem, 140, 270-5
33.   Roels, H, Bernard, A, Buchet, JP, Goret, A, Lauwerys, R,
      Chettle, DR, Harvey, TC and Al Haddad, I (1979).   Critical
      concentration of cadmium in renal cortex and urine. Lancet,
      1, 221
34.   Ellis, KJ, Morgan, WD, Zanzi, I, Yasumura, S, Vartsky, D
      and Cohn, SH (1981).   Critical concentrations of cadmium in
      human renal cortex: dose-effect studies in cadmium smelter
      workers. J Toxicol Environ Hlth, 7, 691-703
35.   Gompertz, D, Chettle, DR, Fletcher, JG, Mason, H, Perkins,
      J Scott, MC, Smith, NJ, Topping, MD and Blindt, M (1983).
      Renal dysfunction in cadmium smelters: Relation to in vivo
      liver and kidney cadmium concentrations. Lancet, 1, 1185-7
36.   Smith, JRH, Athwal, SS, Chettle, DR and Scott, MC (1982).
      On the in vivo measurement of mercury using neutron capture
      and X-ray fluorescence. Int J Appl Radiat Inst, 33, 557-61
37.   Bloch, P and Shapiro, IM (1981).   An X-ray fluorescence
      technique to measure the mercury burden of dentists in vivo.
      Med Phys, 8, 308-11
38.   Knudson, RJ, Slatin, RC, Lebowitz, MD and Burrows, B
      (1976).   The maximal expiratory flow volume curve: Normal
      standards, variability and effects of age. Am Rev Resp Dis,
      113,587-600
39.   Knudson, RJ, Lebowitz, MD, Holberg, CJ, and Burrow, B
      (1983).   Changes in the normal maximal expiratory flow-volume
      curve with growth and ageing. Am Rev Resp Dis, 127, 725-
      34
40.   Ashby, EJ and Richardson, CR (1986).   Tabulation and
      assessment of 113 human surveillance cytogenetic studies con-
      ducted between 1965 and 1984. Mutat Res (In press)
41.   Anderson, D, Richardson, CR, Weight, TM, Purchase, IFH
      and Adams, WGF (1980).   Chromosomal analysis in vinyl

chloride exposed workers. Results from analysis 18 and 42 months after an initial sampling. Mutat Res, 79, 151-62

42. Soper, KA, Stolley, PD, Galloway, SM, Smith, JG, Nichols, WW and Wolman, SR (1984). Sister chromatid exchange (SCE) report on control subjects in a study of occupationally exposed workers. Mutat Res, 129, 77-88

43. Whorton, D, Krauss, RM, Marshall, S and Milby, TH (1977). Infertility in male pesticide workers. Lancet, 2, 1259-61

44. Moore, HDM and Bedford, JM (1983). The interaction of mammalian gametes in the female. In Hartmann, JF (ed.) Mechanism and Control of Animal Fertilization. pp. 453-97. (New York: Academic Press)

45. Edwards, JJ, Tollaksen, SL and Anderson, NG (1981). Proteins of human semen. 1. Two-dimensional mapping of human seminal fluid. Clin Chem, 27, 1335-40

46. Narayan, P, Scott, BK, Millette, CF and De Wolf, WC (1983). Human spermatogenic cell marker proteins detected by two-dimensional electrophoresis. Gamete Res, 7,227-39

47. Hannien, H, Eskelinen, L, Husman, KAJ and Nurminen, M (1976). Behavioural effects of long term exposure to a mixture of organic solvents. Scand J Work Environ Hlth, 2, 240-55

48. Grasso, P, Sharratt, M, Daview, DM and Irvine, D (1984). Neurophysiological and psychological disorders and occupational exposure to organic solvents. Fd Chem Toxicol, 22, 819-52

49. Gilioli, R, Cassitto, MG and Foa, V (eds) (1983). Neurobehavioural Methods in Occupational Health. Advances in the Biosciences, 46. (Oxford: Pergamon Press). Proceedings of the International Symposium on Neurobehavioural Methods in Occupational Health - Como and Milan, June 1982

50. Thompson, WM, Moss, AA and Nelson, JA (1984). Gastrointestinal imaging. Invest Radio, 19, S24-S29

51. Buginger, TF and Lauterbur, PC (1984). Nuclear magnetic resonance technology for medical studies. Science, 226, 288-98

52. Risberg, J and Hagstadius, S (1983). Regional cerebral blood flow by the 133-Xenon inhalation technique. In Gilioli, R, Cassitto, MG and Foa, V (eds) Neurobehavioural Methods in Occupational Health. Advances in the Biosciences, 46, pp. 89-95. (Oxford: Pergamon Press)

53. O'Farrell, PH (1975). High resolution two-dimensional electrophoresis. J Biol Chem, 250, 4007-21

54. Anderson, L and Anderson, N (1984). Some perspectives on two-dimensional protein mapping. Clin Chem, 30, 1898-1905

55. Jellum, E, Orjaseter, H, Harvei, S, Theodorsen, L and Pihl, A (1980). Systematic search for pre-clinical cancer markers in serum: The Janus project. Cancer Detect Prev, 3, Abstract 143

56. Omenn, GS (1982). Predictive identification of hypersusceptible individuals. J Occup Med, 24, 369-74

57. Harrington, JM (1984). Recent Advances in Occupational Health. (London: Churchill Livingstone)

5

Economic Aspects of Toxicity for the Pharmaceutical Industry

G. TEELING SMITH

INTRODUCTION AND HISTORY

This chapter is concerned with the costs of toxicity for the pharmaceutical manufacturers. It does not cover the equally important questions of the costs of toxicity for the individual patient and the health services. It is, however, worth mentioning that these costs are very small compared with the economic benefits created by modern medicines. In economic terms the benefit-risk equation for pharmaceuticals comes out overwhelmingly in favour of the benefit side. The same is, of course, also true for the pharmaceutical manufacturers. At least up to the present, it has remained a profitable business to discover and develop new medicines despite the increasing cost to industry of the consequences of the inevitable toxicity of modern potent medicines.

These growing costs for industry are a relatively new phenomenon. Going back 40 years or so, little attention was paid to the dangers associated with the development and use of medicines. All forms of active medical treatment had well-known risks in the 1930s and before. Surgery was always a risky business because of the elementary nature of the anaesthetic agents available and because of the significant risk of postoperative infection. Against these surgical risks, the dangers of medicines seemed almost insignificant. Hence when it was discovered that penicillin caused some deaths, these were accepted as inevitable. Similarly with the local anaesthetic agent, amethocaine, it was recognized that a young child having a routine tonsillectomy operation might not survive the effects of the anaesthetic, and even diagnostic procedures such as bronchoscopy could be fatal when the same anaesthetic was used.

Yet another example was chloramphenicol. It carried a mortality of about one in 20,000 cases, and this was regarded as an acceptable risk in the 1940s and 1950s. More significantly the antirheumatic preparations, phenylbutazone and oxyphenylbutazone, carried similar risks of fatality; but whereas these risks were accepted at that time, now in the 1980s these medicines have been withdrawn from the market because of their "unacceptable" toxicity. Thus the costs to the industry which are discussed in this chapter have only arisen relatively recently; and they are still increasing, as public concern about the potential toxicity of medicines is being stimulated by consumer organizations throughout the western world.

To a great extent the widespread anxiety about the risks of medication, and hence the consequent costs to the pharmaceutical industry, date back to the thalidomide tragedy in 1961. That event, more than any other, brought home to the public the fact that medicines could do harm as well as good. However, it has been during the 1970s and 1980s that the consumerist pressure groups have greatly increased their activities in publicizing the risks of medicines and in imposing new economic costs on the pharmaceutical industry in consequence. These costs occur in five broad categories, as follows:

1. cost of toxicity testing,
2. delays in marketing while tests continue,
3. costs of postmarketing surveillance for toxic reactions,
4. loss of sales when a medicine is withdrawn,
5. cost of compensation for harm caused.

The rest of this chapter will deal with each of these types of cost in turn.

COST OF TOXICITY TESTING

It was estimated in 1983 that a new medicine costs between £50 million and £90 million to develop, taking into account all the costs of unsuccessful research projects which have to be carried by the few successes actually reaching the market place[1].

Within these total costs of research and development there are various estimates of the amount spent on toxicity testing itself. A large 1984 study by Walker and Prentis[2] from the UK Centre for Medicines Research gives an estimate of 12 per cent of total R and D costs attributable to toxicology. An earlier study in 1979 by Pharma Information in Switzerland[3] gives an estimate of only 6 per cent. It is unlikely that all of the difference is accounted for by an increase in the amount of toxicity testing between 1979 and 1984, but these two studies certainly suggest that the costs are increasing. This testing, of course, consists of animal work, whose significance has to be extrapolated to human experience. The cost of clinical research in the two studies accounted respectively for 18 and 20 per cent of the total. Some proportion of these costs will also be concerned with the investigation of real or apparent toxic reactions during clinical trials.

Given these various estimates it is realistic to suppose that in 1985 a sum of between £5 million and £10 million is spent, on average, on human and animal toxicology for each medicine successfully brought to the market.

DELAYS IN MARKETING

In addition to these direct expenditures on toxicology there are in-
direct costs to the company from sales lost through the delay in
marketing new medicines caused by these tests. It cannot be
argued that it is an imaginary cost because the same eventual earn-
ings are achieved by all medicines a little later than would otherwise be the case. The problem is that the patents on the
medicines expire at a fixed length of time after the medicine has
first been synthesized and the original patent has been filed. In
Europe this is 20 years. In the United States it is 17 years, with
(since 1984) an opportunity to extend this period by up to 5 years
in order to compensate for the delays in the process of getting approval to market the medicine.

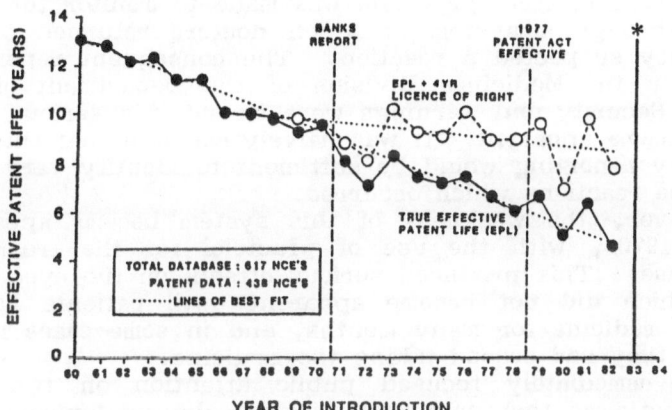

YEAR OF INTRODUCTION

Figure 5.1 The erosion of effective patent life (1960-1982). (From
this point the new chemical entities marketed with the full
20-year patent term will influence the slope of the true effective patent life line)

Figure 5.1 shows the effect on patent life of the lengthening
time which it takes to carry out premarketing tests and to obtain
marketing approval for a new medicine in Britain[4]. The upper
line (with open circles) shows the length of effective patent life
plus 4 years extension (to bring the length of patent to the
present 20 years). The solid black dots show the length of time
left out of an original 16 years of patent life.

Whereas in 1960 under the original 16-year patent a product
still had an effective patent life of 13 years, by 1982, even with a
20-year patent life, the **effective** length of patent protection had
been reduced to 8 years. (On a 16-year patent life little more
than 4 years would have remained). In other words, it now takes
about 12 years between the original synthesis of a new pharmaceutical chemical entity and its first marketing as a medicine.

Much of this delay is due to toxicology, although in some
cases toxicity tests will run in parallel with other development
work. A study by Hartley and Maynard[5] suggested that the
requirements of the 1968 Medicines Act in Britain added 2 years to
the time taken for a new medicine to reach the market. The total

delay due to testing for toxicity probably considerably exceeds this figure.

The economic effect of a shorter period of effective patent protection can be very substantial.   A study by Reekie and Allen[6] has shown that medicines which are subject to generic competition on the expiry of their patent lose market share much faster than those which are still marketed in an exclusive form.

COST OF POSTMARKETING SURVEILLANCE

At the time of the thalidomide tragedy, in 1961, it was presumed that the adverse effects of medicines would usually be spectacular and reasonably easily identifiable.   Nevertheless, in Britain under the 1968 Medicines Act, provision was made to monitor for adverse reactions through a system in which doctors returned a "yellow card" if they suspected a reaction.   The consequent reports were monitored in the Medicines Division of the Department of Health and Social Security and warnings were issued if a serious adverse reaction became apparent.   It was naively assumed that this system of voluntary reporting would be sufficient to identify very quickly any adverse reactions which occurred.

However, the weakness of this system became apparent in the early 1970s, with the use of practolol for the treatment of heart disease.   This produced serious effects on the eyes and the stomach which did not become apparent until patients had been taking the medicine for many months, and in some cases not even until after they had ceased taking the medicine.

This immediately focused public attention on two points. First, it confirmed that no amount of premarketing toxicology could ensure the eventual safety of a medicine.   But second, and more importantly, it pointed up the need to produce more systematic methods of monitoring for adverse reactions in medicines after they have first been marketed.   There was an outcry that "there must never be another practolol", in just the same way as there had previously been an outcry that "there must never be another thalidomide".

The problem is that any method of systematically monitoring the use of every new medicine is extraordinarily expensive.   One extreme forecast (by the author of this chapter) in 1982 predicted that it could cost as much as £55 million per life saved to introduce a fully comprehensive monitoring system to cover every new medicine for its first 3 years on the market[7].   Such enormous costs per life saved arise, of course, because of the extreme rarity of serious adverse effects.

In practice it seems likely that during the 1980s and early 1990s electronic methods of reporting adverse reactions will be introduced, and that the linking of these with computerized systems for monitoring and interpreting the results will reduce costs to a more realistic level.   Nevertheless a comprehensive system of postmarketing surveillance covering all new medicines must be expected to cost sums in the order of millions of pounds per annum in a country such as Britain.

Such expenditures need to be seen in perspective.   They

would probably represent less than 1% of the total pharmaceutical costs. In Britain, again, the amount of money which the government allows companies to spend informing doctors about their new medicines has been reduced by 5% of pharmaceutical sales over the past decade, from 14% to 9%. The consequent savings in expenditure by the companies could therefore have paid for a comprehensive safety monitoring scheme several times over. Other countries could similarly direct parts of their industry's "information" budget to expenditure on safety monitoring.

LOSS OF SALES WHEN MEDICINES ARE WITHDRAWN

So far the costs which have been discussed are incurred in attempting to make medicines as safe in use as possible. The next two types of cost to be discussed are incurred when these safety measures fail, and when - despite all precautions - medicines do in fact do harm.

The first of these two effects comes in loss of sales when a medicine has to be withdrawn. This has become an increasingly common experience during the 1980s, not because medicines have become less safe but because the degree of risk which society will tolerate has been reduced. It has already been pointed out that phenylbutazone and oxyphenylbutazone are excellent examples of this phenomenon.

Table 5.1 Effects of product withdrawal (total of six named products, retail pharmacy purchases, x £1000

Calendar year	Value
1981	11,047
1982	9766
1983	9763
1984	177
1985	0

Note: products included: Butazolidin, Flosint, Opren, Osmosin, Zelmid, Zomax

As a result of these changing attitudes, and increasingly strident demands for a state of affairs approaching absolute safety, eight medicines were withdrawn from the British market during the

83

early 1980s.   Table 5.1 relates to six of these: Butazolidin, Flosint, Opren, Osmosin, Zelmid and Zomax.   It shows the sales of these products year by year over the period when they were withdrawn.   From a figure of sales of over £11 million in 1981 their sales were reduced to zero by 1985.   However even this table understates the degree of loss incurred by the companies concerned. Taking the best calendar years for the sales of each of the six individual products, their total sales would have represented £22.3 million annually.   Although this is little more than 1% of the total pharmaceutical expenditure, the economic impact on the six individual companies which had developed the products was very much greater than that figure indicates.

Each of the companies concerned not only loses the total sales of their product but must write off the cost of existing stocks.   The company has also completely wasted the money it has spent in building up the sales of the product to the moment of its withdrawal.   This is a new hazard, which has become much more evident in the 1980s, and has added substantially to the overall risk of operating in the pharmaceutical business.

COST OF COMPENSATION

Finally, the whole question of compensation for damage caused by medicines is an extremely controversial one.   The legal position in most countries is that a company would only be liable to compensate the sufferer   (or his family) if it could be proved that the manufacturer had been negligent.   In view of the very exhaustive premarketing tests to which a medicine is subjected, it would clearly be extremely difficult ever to prove such negligence.   Companies are meticulous - for their own protection if for no other reason - to ensure that every known precaution is taken to minimize the risk of a medicine for doing harm instead of good.

It has been argued that in consequence the "victim" gets a raw deal, because he cannot validly claim compensation for the harm which has occurred.   This is a matter of continuing debate but, in the meantime, companies are under no legal obligation to compensate those who have suffered for the consequences of genuinely unpredictable adverse reactions.   Nor have they any obligation to pay compensation for predictable damage, provided that proper warnings have been given of known potential adverse reactions.

Nevertheless in practice the situation is very different from this.   Dating back to the experience with thalidomide, there was in that case a violent and prolonged campaign, led by the "Sunday Times" newspaper, to obtain compensation for the victims.   The result was that the British manufacturers paid out over £20 million in compensation for the 400 or so cases of damage caused by the medicine in Britain[8].   That is, an average of about £50,000 per case.

Because the manufacturer had widespread interests outside the pharmaceutical field, it could afford to pay such sums in compensation.   However, had thalidomide and its other pharmaceutical preparations been the company's only source of income, there is little doubt that the compensation payable would have put the company into liquidation.

A similar situation had arisen previously in 1955 in the United States with the Cutter Laboratories' polio vaccine. Although the vaccine in question had passed all the official tests, it nevertheless caused 59 cases of paralytic polio, of which five were fatal. In that case under US law the company was found liable for damages under the rules of warranty, and the company had to pay out over $3 million - $1 million more than its insurance cover[8].

Incidentally, situations such as those experienced with thalidomide cannot be covered by insurance. Because the compensation takes the form of an ex-gratia payment, rather than a legal liability, the insurance company will not accept responsibility.

The case of practolol, which has already been mentioned, also led to substantial payments for ex-gratia compensation, in that case by ICI (once again a large conglomerate company with substantial resources outside its pharmaceutical interests). In that case the company paid compensation to over 1000 people whom it was alleged had been damaged by the medicine. Incidentally the public "bandwagon" effect of offers of compensation is illustrated by the fact that an equal number of claims could be rejected by the company as being unrelated to the use of practolol.

Another case in which unjustifiable claims have been levelled against a company occurred with the much-publicized case of Debendox in the UK and the same medicine sold as Bendectin in the US. Although the authorities, particularly in Britain, have strongly supported the company's view that there is no causal relationship between the use of the medicine during pregnancy and the occurrence of fetal abnormalities, there have been persistent claims for compensation to be paid by the company. These have been rejected in Britain but in the US the company offered an ex-gratia settlement of $120 million, in 1984, rather than incur the cost of defending innumerable individual legal cases. This settlement is still the subject of dispute but its magnitude illustrates the enormous cost which a company can incur when harmful effects are imputed to one of its products - however unjustifiably.

A final example of the escalating cost of compensation for real or alleged harm done by a medicine comes with the case of clioquinol in Japan. Very large numbers of patients claimed that they had been harmed by the medicine, and although some were probably suffering from the effects of other diseases such as multiple sclerosis, the company concerned, Ciba-Geigy, has paid substantial sums in compensation. Up to the end of 1984 these payments had amounted to 500 million Swiss francs, and the company had incurred additional legal and administrative costs of between 50 and 100 million Swiss francs.

PROSPECT FOR THE FUTURE

It seems clear that the costs of toxicology itself, the costs of postmarketing surveillance, and the claims for compensation for alleged adverse effects are all going to continue to increase in the future.

Inevitably this will simply make medicines more expensive than they would otherwise have become. However, the immediate economic consequences of toxicity testing for the pharmaceutical industry are not those which pose the major threat to the continued development of affordable medicines. The actual costs of testing and monitoring for adverse effects will always be a relatively small part of the total cost of developing and marketing a new medicine.

On the other hand, if the situation were to develop unfavourably in respect of compensation for harm done there could be very serious consequences indeed for the pharmaceutical manufacturers and for society as a whole. If the principle of "strict liability" - the right of compensation without any evidence of fault - were to be established either in law, or de facto through consumerist pressures, it could pose a catastrophic threat to individual firms. Claims of thousands of millions of pounds would become possible, and there is no way that most pharmaceutical companies could either insure against such risks or meet such demands from their own resources. Already in the case of clioquinol claims have been in the hundreds of millions of pounds.

The implications of such a situation are already being debated, and there is a strong argument for a major international compensation fund - perhaps with multinational governmental backing through WHO - to meet otherwise impossible demands for compensation. It is in this area that the most significant economic consequences of toxicity in the pharmaceutical field still need to be further considered.

The trend towards a demand for virtually "absolute" safety, and the expectations of automatic massive compensation in any case where this proves to be a chimera, means that pharmaceutical companies could be seriously deterred from putting more investment into the development of much-needed medicines for the still-unconquered disease of today. The only ways to safeguard against this would be either to reverse the trend in public opinion - which is probably impossible - or else to provide realistic financial protection for companies against the risk of otherwise crippling demands for compensation.

As a final note, it should be pointed out that the possibility of an unfavourable balance between potential rewards and potential financial risks in pharmaceutical innovation is not simply a wild theoretical possibility. This situation is already very near to existing in the area of vaccine development. For various economic reasons it is hard to obtain rewarding prices for vaccines and - as in the case of the Cutter polio vaccine - the risk of claims for compensation against vaccine damage are already a common feature. In consequence, very few companies are still putting research funds into the search for new vaccines in the second half of the 1980s.

REFERENCES

1.   Wells, NEJ (1983). Pharmaceutical Innovation. (London: Office of Health Economics)

2. Walker, SA and Prentis, RA (1985). Survey of Research and Development by the UK Pharmaceutical Industry. (London: Centre for Medicines Research)
3. Anonymous (1981). Lifting the Veil on Research. (Basle: Pharma Information)
4. Walker, SA and Prentis, RA (1985). Drug research and pharmaceutical patents. Pharm J, 234, 11-13
5. Hartley, K and Maynard, A (1982). The Costs and Benefits of Regulating New Product Development in the UK Pharmaceutical Industry. (London: Office of Health Economics)
6. Reekie, WD and Allen, DE (1985). Generic substitution in the UK pharmaceutical industry; a Markovian analysis. Manag Decision Econ (In press)
7. Teeling Smith, G (1982). Adverse Reactions and the Community. (London: Office of Health Economics)
8. Teeling Smith, G (1980). A Question of Balance; the benefits and risks of pharmaceutical innovation. (London: Office of Health Economics)

6

Cooperation among States and Setting up an International Legal Framework

J.-M. DEVOS

Safety evaluation of chemicals is an integral part of any environmental policy. Neither as commercial goods, nor as physical substances or preparations can chemicals be isolated from living societies; therefore they cannot escape consideration of policy and law makers. From the commercial viewpoint there has been, particularly since the Second World War, a continuous expansion of international trade in chemicals, especially among industrialized countries.

Naturally, chemicals are sometimes distributed in the environment over great distances through air or water conductors. The evaluation of the potential effects of chemicals, their impact on human health and safety and their action on the whole environment is therefore a common legitimate worry to industrialists and scientists, but also to the public, particularly through the public authorities responsible for safeguarding or protecting the general public. This preoccupation cannot be limited to a district, province, region or even country. More and more environmental protection in its wide sense calls for international cooperation.

This article sets out to describe what have been the previous efforts and what are the prospects for international cooperation and harmonization in the specific context of the control of chemicals and their safety evaluation.

International cooperation in the western world, advanced actions has been undertaken by the OECD[n1] and the EC[n2]. Both organizations are basically oriented towards economic development through international cooperation, though in the case of the EC the process is oriented towards real integration.

While economic growth and industrial development have clearly received priority in the 1950s and 1960s, the end of the 1960s has seen a reconsideration of the problems raised by the development of advanced societies. The new political dimension of environmental issues led to the launching of programmes which in their initial phases contained declarations of intentions with few practical or effective results. However, the structure of specialized cooperation and policy-making bodies was progressively created. In 1970 came the formation of the OECD Environment

Committee. This Committee was established by all member countries to form various working bodies including "the chemicals group". Another significant step was achieved when a "Management Committee for the Special Programme on the Control of Chemicals" was created in 1979, reporting directly to the OECD Council, but not representing all OECD member countries. Representatives of the EC, and observers from other international organizations such as the specialized agencies of the UN system, take part in meetings in order to ensure harmonization of work at international level[n3].

Expert groups and working parties have been created by these policy-making bodies, where member countries nominate experts from their public or private sectors. Business, industry and trade unions are often involved through their recognized bodies.

The European Communities' objectives under the Treaty of Rome are basically oriented towards economic integration and free movement of goods, persons and services. The Treaty of Rome contains no specific provision relating to environment protection or policy. However, since 1972 a political consensus appeared at the level of the member states, which recognized the need to develop community action in the area of environmental protection. This led to the adoption in November 1973 by the Council of Ministers of the first action programme[1], which has since been renewed in 1977[2] and 1983[3]. The reasons for taking action at Community level were based on economic and environmental considerations. Firstly, as the Rome Treaty is directed towards economic integration and the creation of a vast, united internal market, it was assumed that differences in environmental policy could lead to distortions of competition. Secondly, there was a growing political awareness that the Community could not ignore such an important dimension of its population's well-being. Remarkable achievements have been realized in a 10-year period, as more than 100 legal instruments were adopted, including important directives on the control of chemicals.

Alongside the development of major environmental action by inter-governmental organizations such as the OECD, or supranational bodies such as the EC, industry was more and more made aware of the need to deal with environmental problems at international level. In order to pursue a necessary dialogue with the public authorities who were in charge of defining the new policies, organizations such as the European Council of Chemical Manufacturers Federations (CEFIC) were created in the early 1970s with the declared objective to seek solutions on problems relating to international collaboration, etc. Other bodies such as the Business and Industry Advisory Committee (BIAC) and the Trade Unions Advisory Committee (TUAC) have been involved in activities relating to the OECD programmes on chemicals.

THE OECD PROGRAMME ON CHEMICALS

The OECD member countries decided to complement and harmonize their national legislative and regulatory activities related to the protection of man and the environment from risks associated with chemicals. This programme had four main objectives:

1. to improve the protection of health and the environment from harmful effects of chemicals;
2. to avoid distortions of trade in chemicals;
3. to reduce the economic and administrative burden on member countries associated with chemicals control;
4. to foster international exchange of information on chemicals.

The chemicals group created by the Environment Committee focused its initial work on a few chemicals known for having already caused contamination problems. Reports were prepared on polychlorinated biphenyls (PCBs), mercury and cadmium. A decision on the restriction of use of PCBs was adopted by the OECD Council in 1973[4]. This decision was the first international attempt to control the environmental hazards of a specific chemical. A recommendation restricting mercury emmissions was adopted in the same year[5]. The chemicals group monitored developments in PCBs and mercury in the member countries but also extended its activity to other products such as chlorofluorocarbons (CFCC).

GENERAL CONTROL OF CHEMICALS AND COOPERATION WITHIN OECD

From 1973 it became clear that there was a strong need to develop procedures to assess the potential hazard of chemicals before their entry onto the market. Purely national policies in this area could have brought economic distortions in the circulation of goods, and disruption of international trade. This common awareness led to the adoption of the OECD Council Recommendation of 14 November 1974[6]. The adoption of this recommendation represented a major step forward on the road to consistent international cooperation for the general control of chemicals. The 1974 Recommendation provided the legal basis for the OECD's activities in this area.

On the basis of various investigations relating, among other things, to pre-market scrutiny, ways of controlling chemicals and safety testing[7], the OECD Council adopted a further Recommendation which provided procedures for assessing chemicals[8]. In the international approach to chemicals assessment, mutual acceptability of information, and therefore of testing methods, were recognized as priority actions. This led to the 1977 OECD Chemicals Testing Programme.

The aim was to develop internationally recognized guidelines which would indicate how testing should be carried out. This required extensive studies on the evaluation of the state of art in testing chemical properties needed to assess the potential hazards of a chemical to man or the environment. Testing methods for physical and chemical properties, environmental degradation and accumulation potential, short- and long-term toxicity, and ecotoxicity were studied. The concept of "step-sequence" testing was also examined from the consideration of an initial assessment of a chemical (minimum data set) to criteria for developing more complex and therfore costly testing.

THE SPECIAL PROGRAMME ON THE CONTROL OF CHEMICALS

In addition to the work undertaken in the Chemicals Testing Programme, other priority areas were defined in the framework of the "Special Programme on the Control of Chemicals". This programme was adopted in 1978[9] as a response to the need for stronger international cooperation in view of the chemical laws due to be adopted in various OECD countries or areas, such as the European Communities "Sixth amendment" on the US "Toxic Substance Control Act". The special programme covered four main topics:

(a) Good laboratory practice ("GLP"). The objective was to prepare a set of principles governing how laboratory testing facilities should be managed to ensure proper testing and quality control. Such a joint approach led to the consideration of means for harmonizing national procedures. This would enable member countries to recognize each other's test data as generated according to internationally accepted procedures.

(b) Confidentiality of data and control of chemicals. An essential aspect of the confidence required for the proper functioning of reciprocal data exchange was the status of commercially sensitive information. It was therefore essential to ensure that proprietary rights on data submitted by the industry would be protected in an appropriate manner and would be equally guaranteed by the Member Countries.

(c) International glossary of terms. The idea of this action was to develop a consistent terminology of the key terms which are used in chemicals control legislation. Common or similar concepts and definitions were essential in any serious attempt to harmonize more legislation.

(d) Information exchange procedures. Activities on exchange procedures between member countries were studied by the OECD secretariat and covered, among other things, the exchange between member countries of information on the development in new laws legislation.

ACHIEVEMENTS OF THE OECD PROGRAMME, AND ADOPTION OF INTERNATIONALLY BINDING INSTRUMENTS

Quite remarkably, in about 10 years, the OECD chemicals programme led to the adoption of various international acts which had a direct impact on the member country policies.

The OECD Council, which is the main body of the organization where all member countries are represented at ministerial or permanent representative level, endorsed various proposals made at the First High Level Meeting of the Chemicals Group (HLM I in May 1980) and at the Second High Level Meeting of the Chemicals Group (HLM II in November 1982).

MUTUAL ACCEPTANCE OF DATA AND ASSESSMENT OF CHEMICALS

The Council adopted a Decision on the Mutual Acceptance of Data[10]. The decision is based on the principle that if test data have been generated in one OECD member country in accordance with the OECD Test Guidelines and the OECD Principles of Good Laboratory Practice, these data have to be accepted by the other OECD member countries as valid for use in assessment procedures, and in any other uses relating to the protection of man and of the environment. The advantages of such a rule are obvious. Test data obtained in one OECD member country in accordance with the OECD principles on test guidelines and good laboratory practice ought not to be repeated or reproduced in the other countries. This should bring a sharp reduction in testing and assessment costs and thus foster international trade in chemicals.

The decision was therefore followed by two related recommendations to use the OECD Test Guidelines and to apply the OECD Principles of Good Laboratory Practice (GLP). The Council adopted a number of Test Guidelines and a mechanism of updating in the light of scientific progress was agreed[11].

The expert group on Good Laboratory Practice completed its work in 1982, which led to the publication of a report[12]. The principles of GLP recommended by the group were described in chapter 2 of this report. They dealt with the modes of organizing studies and conditions relating to the planning, realization, control, registration and diffusion of laboratory studies. In 1983 the OECD Council adopted a Recommendation on the Mutual Recognition of Compliance with Good Laboratory Practice[13]. The implementation of GLP by the OECD member states and by the EEC has become more and more effective.

The work on Test Guidelines has been and still is continued in the "Updating Programme". Existing Test Guidelines are reviewed in the light of scientific and technological progress. The Updating Panel, supported by experts from the member countries, prepares revisions and new Test Guidelines. The harmonized assessment of testing results is the logical follow-up of harmonized testing. Consequently, Provisional Data Interpretation Guides have been published in relation with the OECD guidelines for testing chemicals.

Finally, in the wake of a statement made during the Second High Level Meeting of the Chemicals Group, the Updating Panel is considering the possible revision of existing Test Guidelines which would minimize the use of animals in laboratory testing.

OTHER LEGISLATIVE ACHIEVEMENTS

After the Second High Level Meeting of the OECD, the OECD Council adopted various acts, i.e.

1. Decision on the Minimum Premarket set of Data ("MPD")[14]. This decision established the regime applicable to the new chemicals to be put on the market. The principle is that

sufficient information on the properties of chemicals should be made available before they are marketed.

2.   Three Recommendations linked to the important issue of the protection of rights of the owner of the information were adopted in July 1983[15-17].

THE EC AND THE LEGISLATION ON PREVENTIVE
CONTROL OF CHEMICALS

In parallel to the progress and harmonization efforts achieved in the OECD context, the EC has developed a set of legal instruments in relation to the control of chemicals. The most significant of these instruments in the so-called "Sixth Amendment", actually a Community Directive amending a 1967 Directive on Dangerous Substances[18]. "The Sixth Amendment" established a system of premarketing notification and assessment of new chemical substances. It also defined packaging and labelling conditions.

The system is based on the obligation imposed on the producer or importer of a chemical product in the EC territory to notify to the national competent authority a technical dossier, a declaration on the unfavourable effects of the substance, a proposal for classification and labelling, and proposals for any recommended precautions relating to the safe use of the substance. This notification must take place at the latest 45 days before introduction into the market. The dossier submitted to the competent authorities of one member state is transmitted to the Commission and, through this Institution, to the other member states. The notification is therefore valid in all member states and premarketing notification and testing is no longer necessary in the various individual countries. Though initially addressed to the authorities of one member state, the notification has clearly a community character. The notification requirements apply to all chemicals marketed for the first time after 18 September 1981. Logically, the directive had to develop harmonized solutions for the tests to be carried out and the assessment methods (physicochemical properties, toxicity and ecotoxicity).

In order to preserve the legitimate property rights of the notifier, the directive also provides for a system of protection of confidential data which guarantees secrecy of commercially sensitive information. Secrecy is guaranteed versus any person other than the competent authorities and the Commission. A limited amount of data cannot benefit from confidential treatment, i.e. the trade name of the substance, various physicochemical data concerning the substance, the possible ways of rendering the substance harmless, the interpretation of the toxicological and ecotoxicological tests and the name of the reponsible laboratory, the recommended methods and precautions.

The directive is now in its implementation phase, and though many difficulties must still be expected in applying the system, it is clear today that the sixth amendment represents a major integrated and supranational system of chemicals control. The next step   will be the definition of a community regime applicable to dangerous preparations[n4].

CASE LAW OF THE EC COURT OF JUSTICE, AND ACTION OF THE EUROPEAN COMMISSION

The case law of the EC Court of Justice on articles 30 to 36 of the Rome Treaty has also contributed indirectly to the progress of mutual recognition of data and tests. These provisions are related to the free circulation of goods. Articles 30 to 34 prohibit "quantitative restrictions on imports and all measures having equivalent effect". Article 36 admits, however, that prohibitions or restrictions to the free movement of goods may be justified, i.e. on grounds of protection of health and life of humans, animals or plants.

The Court of Justice has given some precisions from the limits of the powers of the EC member states in the area. To be accepted, national rules derogating to the principle of free circulation have to satisfy a mandatory requirement, being necessary and proportional to the purpose served. In its "Frans-Nederlandse Maatschappij voor Biologische Produkten" case[19], the Court recognized the right of the states to require approval procedures prior to the entry of a pesticide into their territory when health protection aspects were involved.

However, states may not needlessly require chemical analyses or tests where the same analyses or tests had already been carried out, and where their results might be placed at their disposal. While the states retained a supervisory power, they were obliged to take account of what had already been done in another member state. As far as the condition of similarity of tests and analyses were concerned, the reference ought to be made to the objective and to the purpose of analyses rather than to their possible technical differences.

It is interesting to note that the conclusions reached by the Court, though based on different legal provisions, were going in the same direction as the orientations mentioned above in the regulatory activities of the OECD and the EEC. In its 1985 "White Paper"[20] on the internal market, the Commission of the European Communities declared that it would use all the powers available under the Treaty, particularly articles 30-36, to reinforce the principle of mutual recognition.

In the specific area of testing and certification procedures the Commission declared its intention to take an initiative involving the drawing-up of common conditions and codes of practice for implementation by laboratories and certification bodies. Such codes would be based on existing codes of Good Laboratory Practice and Good Manufacturing Practice already widely used. The Commission has adopted a proposal for a directive on the application of principles of Good Laboratory Practice and control of their application for testing of chemical substances[21]. This proposal obliges laboratories carrying out tests under the community legislation on chemicals to certify that the tests have been made in accordance with the principles of Good Laboratory Practice specified in Annex 2 of the OECD Decision of 12 May 1981 on the Mutual Acceptance of

THE FUTURE OF PREDICTIVE SAFETY EVALUATION

Data in the Assessment of Chemicals.

CONCLUSION

The example of the "Sixth Amendment" and the progress achieved in the OECD Chemical Programme will, without any doubt, influence any new attempts to define international solutions to the transboundary problem of controlling chemicals and ensuring at the same time their free circulation. From a broader standpoint there is no doubt that the development of issues such as toxicology and restricting the use of animals in testing will have to be solved through international mechanisms, and through the necessary cooperation between the scientific community, the industry and national or supranational authorities[n5].

NOTES

[n1] The Organization for European Economic Cooperation was established in 1948, originally in order to promote cooperation between the European countries under the Marshall Plan. Today it provides a forum for 24 industrialized countries from North America, Western Europe, Asia and Oceania.

[n2] European Communities. Originally founded in 1957 under the Treaty of Rome. Its membership is open to European countries and totalled 12 countries in January 1986.

[n3] This article does not cover activities existing at the UN level in bodies like the United Nations Environment Programme (UNEP), the International Labour Organization (ILO) and the World Health Organization (WHO).

[n4] The EEC Commission has presented in the course of the month of July 1985 a proposal for a Council Directive on the approximation of the laws regulations and administrative provisions of the member states relating to the classification, packaging and labelling of dangerous preparations (Doc. COM(85) 36 (final)).

[n5] In its draft resolution on a programme of action of the European Communities on toxicology for health protection (Official Journal of the EC no. C 156/6 (16.6.1984), the EC Commission reaffirmed the need to ensure the quality and comparability of toxicological data and of testing methods. To prevent duplication of efforts, cooperation with organizations of the UN and the OECD was deemed essential in areas such as research, setting up equivalent standards for the training of toxicologists, reduction of animal experiments and

harmonization of assessment criteria concerning substances which are dangerous to health.

REFERENCES

1. Declaration of 22 November 1973 of the Council of the European Communities and of the Representatives of the Governments of the member states meeting in the Council on the Action Programme of the European Communities on the Environment. Official Journal of the EC no. C.112 (20.12.73)
2. Resolution of 15 May 1977 of the Council of the European Communities and of the Representatives of the Governments of the member states meeting in the Council on the Continuation and Implementation of a European Community Policy and Action Programme on the Environment. Official Journal of the EC no. C.139 (13.6.77)
3. Resolution of 7 February 1983 of the Council of the European Communities and of the Representatives of the Governments of the member states meeting within the Council on the continuation and implementation of a European Community Policy and Action Programme on the Environment (1982-1986) Official Journal of the EC no. C.46 (7.2.83)
4. Decision of 13 February 1973 on Protection of the Environment by Control of Polychlorinated Biphenyls (C(73) 1 (final))
5. Recommendation of 18 September 1973 on Measures to Reduce all Man-Made Emissions of Mercury to the Environment (C(73) 172 (final))
6. Recommendation on the Assessment of the Potential Environmental Effects of Chemicals (C(74) 215 (final))
7. Regulations relating to environmental control of chemicals: premarket and postmarket controls, Paris (1976); Chemical assessment: Industry's Approach to Safety Testing, OECD, Paris (1976)
8. Recommendations of 7 July 1977 establishing guidelines in respect of procedures and requirements for anticipating the effects of chemicals on man in the environment (C(77) 97 (final))
9. Decision of 21 September 1979 on a Special Programme on the Control of Chemicals (C(78) 127 (final))
10. Decision of 12 May 1981 on the Mutual Acceptance of Data in the Assessment of Chemicals (C(81) 30 (final))
11. OECD guidelines for Testing of Chemicals (1981 and continuing series)
12. Good Laboratory Practice in the Testing of Chemicals, OECD, Paris (1982)
13. Recommendation of 26 July 1983 on Mutual Recognition of Compliance with Good Laboratory Practice (C(83) 95 (final))
14. Decision of 8 December 1982 on the Minimum Pre-marketing Set of Data in the Assessment of Chemicals (C(82) 196 (final))
15. Recommendation of 26 July 1983 on the Exchange of Confiden-

tial Data on Chemicals (C(83) 97 (final))
16. Recommendation of 26 July 1983 on Protection of Proprietary Rights to Data Submitted in Notification of New Chemicals (C(83) 96 (final))
17. Recommendation of 26 July 1983 on the OECD list of Non-Confidential Data on Chemicals (C(83) 98 (final))
18. Directive 79/831/EEC of 18 September 1979 amending for the sixth time Directive 67/548/EEC on the approximation of the laws, regulations and administrative provisions relating to the classification, packaging and labelling of dangerous substances. Official Journal of the EC no. L.259 (15.10.79)
19. Decision of the Court of 17 December 1981 (272/80)
20. Completing the Internal Market, White paper from the Commission of the European Council (Milan, 28-29 June 1985) (Dec. COM(85) 310 (final))
21. Proposal for a Directive presented by the Commission to the EC Council on 24 July 1985 (COM(85) 380 final, published in the Official Journal of the EC no. C.219 (29.8.1985))

PART 2
The Needs
(Non-pharmaceutical)

7
Foods and Food Additives

D. M. CONNING AND K. R. BUTTERWORTH

The toxicology of food has always been a science divided between two laudable objectives. The first and most ancient objective is the essentially practical one of defining what is safe to eat. It seems likely that even primitive man learned to define good foods and bad foods by observation of animals, and by associating taste with adverse responses such as bitterness or nausea. This aspect of toxicology finds its counterpart today in the regulatory control of the quality of foodstuffs using more advanced methods. The second objective is to understand the mechanism whereby a chemical adversely affects biological systems. The purpose of this is as much to understand about the functioning of the biological system as to define the toxic mechanism. Safety considerations have increasingly overshadowed, and currently almost eclipsed, the investigations of the mechanisms of production of any toxic effects produced by food.

Apart from substantial safeguards for animal health, the major consideration in all regulatory systems is the protection of human health. Initially regulations were devised in an attempt to curb the fraudulent contamination of foodstuffs. Latterly the controls have developed in relation to advances in food technology and the increasing number of compounds used in food processing.

Toxicological studies recognize essentially two variables - dose and duration of administration. These variables arise from two basic observations. First that the severity of an effect is usually related directly to the amount of compound administered. Secondly, compounds administered repeatedly, even at small dosage, for long periods of time (e.g. lifetime studies in experimental rats) can result in disease processes such as cancer or the failure of an organ system.

During the first half of this century the development of these studies resulted in a formal system of testing eventually incorporated into practical manuals so much used that the procedures have become enshrined as classic. Regrettably such studies still use as their endpoints the identification of "effects", with no attempt to elucidate the mechanism whereby the effect is produced. It is often the case that the effect itself is assumed to be abnormal

101

because the authorities, recognizing the extent of ignorance concerning the mechanisms of biological function, judged it impossible to ascertain when a given observation of effect could be defined as within the normal physiological response. It was decided therefore that assessments of safety would be related to the detection of any effect resulting from the treatment of an experimental animal with a chemical compound. Where more than one species was examined the results in the most sensitive species would be used - that is that dose just below the smallest dose to produce an effect irrespective of species, would be employed in the subsequent calculations. This dosage is known as the "no-effect level" (NEL). It is usually divided by a "safety" factor ranging from 100 to 1000 to give the acceptable daily intake (ADI), expressed as an amount per unit body weight per day. The ADI is deemed to be the dosage that may be consumed daily by adult man for life without untoward effect. The safety factor of 100 is said to be based on a tenfold reduction to take account of possible differences in species sensitivity and a further tenfold factor to take account of human heterogeneity. Higher factors may be used but the criteria have never been defined. They often depend on the judgement of the assessor.

As a consequence of the rapid increase of biological knowledge, and of the increasingly sensitive analytical techniques, the derivation of NELs has required a very substantial increase of the data collected in toxicological experiments. Similarly the development of statistical techniques has usually resulted in the use of more experimental animals. The consequence has been a regulatory demand for enormous amounts of data, covering many biological fields, when new compounds are to be incorporated into the human diet or environment. These data are usually not relevant to mechanisms of toxicity and therefore have added little to the understanding of toxicological processes. Further, their acquisition has diverted enormous effort away from toxicological research, so that there has been little advance in our understanding of such mechanisms. As a consequence the prediction of human safety remains empirical, based on observations in the experimental animal with the assumption that man responds similarly.

The system appears to have been effective in protecting public health in that there are a few authentic instances of illness associated with food chemicals used normally, though there have been several examples of accidental poisoning. The possibility that food chemicals have induced adverse effects in man comes closest to realization in respect of potential immunological sensitization. Although it has proved difficult to identify specific antibody production, the clinical presentations of reactions to, for example, sulphur dioxide or tartrazine are suggestive. The absence of an animal model as sensitive as the human immune system has proved a handicap in the investigation of such effects.

In general, whether the regulatory procedures have protected the public health cannot be proved because none of the studies commonly employed can with certainty predict the nature of the human response or the degree of human sensitivity, and no attempts have been made to assess the efficacy of regulatory control on human disease patterns. It seems a possibility that the absence of toxic effects may be due to the low concentrations of food additives used in food technology, rather than the assay of toxicological hazard and the setting of an ADI.

FUTURE PROBLEMS IN FOOD TOXICOLOGY

Such problems may be classified as either methodological or related to the type of product to be evaluated.

Methodological

There are two continuing problems in the evaluation of food and food chemicals, and it is a matter of regret that they persist despite the amount of testing undertaken in recent decades. The first concerns the prediction of human hazard from the results of animal experiments; the second the prediction of long-term effects on the basis of relatively short-term trials.

The process of inter-species extrapolation has shown marked advance in respect of comparative metabolism in that it is common practice to compare metabolic activity in several species. Such studies usually show that there is a qualitative similarity between species but there are marked quantitative differences. It is often the case that a number of metabolic pathways exist which vary in significance in different species. The preferred pathway depends on the individual species and may be relevant to the toxicity of the substance in that species. For example, coumarin is metabolized by a number of different pathways in various species[1]. Since the rat metabolizes coumarin quite differently from man, the suitability of the rat as a test species in predicting the hepatotoxic risk to man has been questioned. Whether coumarin or a metabolite is the active hepatotoxin has not been established with certainty. However, the evidence so far obtained suggests that the metabolic pathway is an important factor in determining the hepatotoxic response, and therefore species differences in metabolism should be taken into account in evaluating the hepatotoxic hazard to man.

The second problem is, in part, the relevance of the relative life spans of, for example, rat and man, and whether the discrepancy (2-3 years against 60-70 years respectively) has a biological basis that is important to the interpretation of toxic effects. Such a basis clearly exists for metabolic rate, which can be standardized in relation to bodyweight or surface area, and it may be assumed that such a basis exists for standardizing all biological activity.

Another aspect of this problem is the relationship that exists between short-term effects and long-term consequences. Chronic toxic effects may arise in three ways. First, the relentless burden of dealing with foreign materials consistently present in the diet may lead to a diminution of the reactive response and the eventual expression of a toxic effect. This diminution of a defensive response might itself occur as an effect of age. For example, it is known that hepatomas induced by the colour Ponceau MX in the young rat develop into hepatocellular carcinomas as the animal ages[2]. Second, short-term exposure may have an effect on gene expression that eventually results in a recognizable disease process. This is thought to be the basis of genotoxic carcinogenesis. Benzpyrene, which occurs in various refined, broiled and smoked foods, is an example of this process[3]. Again the effect may occur as a result of the interaction of many factors such as age, the presence of promoters, sex hormones etc. Third, the long-continued presence of the foreign material causes a chronic toxic effect directly. An example here might be hypercarotenaemia induced by the excessive ingestion of raw carrots by man[4]. It is very unlikely that extrapolation from animal to man can be meaningful unless the animal model exhibits a range of chronic disease syndromes comparable to that of man.

The only approach to safety assessment that is likely to offer improvement in respect of these problems is that based on an understanding of the toxicological mechanisms and the determination of whether those mechanisms can operate in man. It may not be necessary, in this regard, to know the precise molecular mechanism. It may suffice to know only the biochemical system involved or the primary organelle affected. Thus in human medicine it is often possible to characterize clinical syndromes by changes in blood chemistry without knowing the precise mechanism whereby the changes arise. Similarly it may be possible to characterize toxicological response in one species with sufficient precision to be able to suggest whether such an effect could occur in another species. This approach would require the following investigative stages:

1. A careful pharmacokinetic study to define absorption and excretion, tissue distribution and concentration of the active substance, principal metabolites, target organ toxicity and, by ultrastructural examination, a definition of the organelles affected in the cellular dysfunction which is the basis of the aberrrant response. Such studies may require elucidation of the effects of the intestinal flora and may involve pharmacological rather than morphologal analysis.

2. Culture studies of the target organ tissue in which biochemical analysis of the damaged cells is undertaken, utilizing the dose of the chemical or metabolite determined by the pharmacokinetic study. The purpose of this phase would be to elucidate the principal enzyme changes (inhibitions or deletions) that were associated with the dysfunction. Such studies would not amount to elucidation of total toxic mechanisms but to identification of key effects consistently associated with observed changes.

3. Repetition of the culture studies using human tissues to determine whether the effects associated with the toxic consequences could be reproduced, and the determination of the critical doses involved.

Such an approach would relate the observed effects to a realistic dosage in relation to the intended use of the compound, and would avoid errors introduced by gross overdosage, such as that achieved by a "maximum tolerated dose" approach. It would allow extrapolations to man to be based on common observations in the experimental model and the human equivalent. It would deal with the compounds pertinent to the observed effect, which may be metabolites, and not rely on possibly fallacious assumptions attributed to the parent compound. Finally it would provide data on toxicological mechanisms rather than statements of the effects produced.

The main disadvantage to such an approach is that associated with any scientific investigation, namely that the biochemical approach would have to be very broad to avoid missing effects. This disadvantage is reduced by the emphasis on key effects rather than on all effects, but could be further reduced by the following additional activities. Structure-activity assessments would enable certain potential effects to be identified before investigations began, (e.g. polycyclic hydrocarbons may be carcinogenic[5]). The studies could with advantage be confined, as a first priority, to those systems known to be affected by the common chronic ailments of man. The rationale of this is that significant chronic chemical poisoning is most likely to manifest itself as a chronic degenerative condition of a type commonly seen in man.

The prediction of potential carcinogenic effects would depend on the now conventional genotoxic studies with metabolic activation (e.g. use of S9 liver fraction in the Ames Test[6]). These test systems based on modified bacteria can show major defects in the prediction of carcinogenic potential of compounds not previously tested, in that materials which are carcinogenic in animal studies are not necessarily detected in bacterial mutation assays[7,8] (e.g. benzene, asbestos, diethylstilboestrol, di-2-ethylhexyl phthalate). This is less so with mammalian cell systems or tests involving in vivo studies such as the induction of chromosomal abnormalities in bone marrow. A negative result in such studies could be taken to indicate an absence of genotoxic potential. A positive result would probably lead to the abandonment of the development on the grounds of potential mutagenicity or possibly to more extensive (and expensive) analyses.

There has been a recent revival of the concept of tumour promotion, and it seems likely that some assay of this potential will be required. Many of the developments of the concepts of growth factors show considerable promise although their translation from the culture dish to the living animal has yet to be achieved. It is likely that this problem will be solved by the burgeoning efforts on gene control of cell proliferation.

In the longer term it is to be expected that toxicological studies, particularly of dietary components as opposed to additives, will need to take account of the genetic susceptibility of the individual. It is already clear, for example, that the adverse effects of saturated fat or salt, if they exist at all, must be related in part to the genetic susceptibility of the consumer. In future it is to be hoped that personal advice on proper dietary control will be related to a better understanding of the requirements of the individual, so avoiding wholesale manipulation of nutrient intake because of a susceptible minority.

Such developments will embrace the concept of human monitoring, and it is certainly important that such concepts are introduced for public debate in order to prevent the ethical issues being sidetracked by emotional harangues.

New products

Over the coming decades there is likely to be a marked increase in the products coming from biotechnological developments. These will arise from the identification and isolation of organisms with particular characteristics but also from the impact of genetic engineering in a wide variety of applications. Many of these developments will result in compounds used extensively in food processing or as dietary components; or indeed as complete foods if the genetic manipulation of plants is considered.

Care will be needed to ensure that the byproducts of growth under certain conditions (myco- and bacterial toxins) are detectable and detected. It is possible that such products will incorporate compounds such as branched-chain fatty acids not normally encountered in human diet, and the possible adverse consequences will need to be detected. In genetically engineered products some safeguards against residual abnormal DNA capable of being transfected will be needed. At present the only methods available to guard against such eventualities are those dependent on detailed chemical analysis. For the immediate future it is likely that products containing residual DNA or abnormal fatty acids will need to be excluded. A conventional approach to safety evaluation based on animal studies is unlikely to be cost-effective or scientifically feasible.

Miscellaneous problems

Finally there may be a number of food safety problems related to newly identified syndromes. The contemporary concern with food sensitivity and food intolerance is an example of a clinical syndrome for which there is as yet no satisfactory scientific explanation and yet which appears susceptible to treatment. Such observations suggest that it is possible that certain behavioural abnormalities hitherto considered to be psychoneurotic in origin could be due to as yet undefined reactions against dietary components, though it remains the case that no objective evidence exists to support this contention. It is important that such evidence should be accumulated rapidly. This is particularly important in the case of the maladjustment or hyperactive syndromes of childhood where dietary manipulation appears to have achieved good results in a few refractory cases[9,10].

Nevertheless it is now certain that many of the heritable metabolic deficiency syndromes are present in the "normal" population at much less penetration due to gene dilution. If this is the case it is certainly conceivable that some disease entities occur with greater frequency where there is an inherited susceptibility will be a further task for the molecular biologist. The recognition of dietary components likely to provide such reactions is a problem to tax the minds of future generations of toxicologists.

REFERENCES

1. Cohen, AJ (1979). Critical review of the toxicology of coumarin with special reference to interspecies differences in metabolism and hepatotoxic response and their significance to man. Fd Cosmet Toxicol, 17, 277-89
2. Grasso, P and Gray, TJB (1977). Long-term studies on chemically induced liver enlargement in the rat. III. Structure and behaviour of the hepatic nodular lesions induced by Ponceau MX. Toxicology, 7, 327-47
3. Lintas, C, de Matthaeis, MC and Merli, F (1979). Determination of Benzol[α]pyrene in smoked, cooked and toasted food products. Fd Cosmet Toxicol, 17, 325-8
4. Sharman, IM (1985). Hypercarotenaemia. Br Med J, 290, 95-6
5. IARC Monographs (1983). The evaluation of the carcinogenic risk of chemicals to humans. Vol. 32. Polynuclear Aromatic Compounds, Part 1, Chemical, Environmental and Experimental Data. (Lyon: World Health Organization)
6. Ames, BN, McCann, J and Yamasuki, E (1975). Methods for detecting carcinogens and mutagens with the Salmonella/mammalian-microsome mutagenicity test. Mutation Res, 31, 347-64
7. Ashby, J, de Serres, FJ, Draper, M, Ishidate, M Jr, Margolin, BH, Matter, BE and Shelby, MD (eds) (1985). Evaluation of short-term tests for carcinogens. Report of the International Programme on Chemical Safety's Collaborative Study on in vitro Assays Progress in Mutation Res, Vol 5, pp. 117-74 (Amsterdam: Elsevier Science Publishers)
8. Sobels, FH (1985). Editorial. A comprehensive exercise in comparative mutagenesis with exciting outcome - or - How good are mutation assays in predicting carcinogens? Mutation Res, 147, 1-4
9. Egger, J, Carter, CM, Graham, PJ, Gumley, D and Soothill, JF (1985). Controlled trial of oligoantigenic treatment in the hyperkinetic syndrome. Lancet, 1, 540-5
10. Tryphonas, H and Trites, R (1984). Diet and hyperactivity. BNF Nutr Bull, 9, 24-31

8

Industrial Chemicals

M. A. COOKE

The past decade has seen a world wide proliferation of legislation intended to protect the worker and the public against any ill-effects of exposure to industrial chemicals. It is often assumed that more tests will result in greater safety and that harmonization of test protocols will render the results of tests more readily acceptable to others. The harmonization effected by OECD guidelines[1] has assisted in the institution of minimal standards, but whether increased legislation has increased ultimate safety to any significant degree is more debatable and the overall cost to the community has barely been considered. Of even greater importance is the consideration whether the funding could not have been more profitably and efficiently applied to individually prepared programmes and protocols linked to specific chemicals and their perceived risks.

In some cases a more liberal self-regulatory approach is evident, as in the requirements for premarketing notification (PMN) under the Toxic Substances Control Act (TSCA) of the USA, where toxicity data are not essential to the notification, although clearly the Environmental Protection Agency have powers to require specific reassurance or testing as indicated. In a similar fashion the Occupational Safety and Health Administration (OSHA) have moved towards consideration of managements' total systems for health and safety maintenance, and provides for exemption for certain general inspections for approved employers[2].

In Europe, on the other hand, we see increased attention to detailed legislation and toxicity testing requirements for both new and existing chemicals. With the advent of a "Preparations Directive" this will become even more onerous, increasing production costs and areas of uncertainty without necessarily minimizing any current or future risks.

The cost of testing is a not inconsiderable item. Commercial testing houses have proliferated as a result of legislation and general demand in the past 30 years, and increasing competition, have resulted in more sophisticated units with a capability for more intricate studies. The interpretations of the results of such studies often raise their own problems and may increase both total cost and uncertainty - perhaps the best examples of this are current genotoxicity tests. Few give a definitive answer as far as ultimate safety is concerned.

However, the mere expression of the weakness of our current system is a negative approach to be deplored, and a positive approach to render our total environment the safer must be our aim. Safety of product and of manufacturing processes is in the best long-term interest of any manufacturer, and investment in a sound safety evaluation programme within an equally sound total health and safety programme produces greater return, both short- and long-term, than is sometimes appreciated.

What then should be our aims and strategies in the next decade and in the longer term? I would suggest our principal aims should be:

1. The maintenance at least, and more desirably a steady improvement, of our current hazard awareness, safety evaluation and toxicity testing and the implementation of adequate health and safety programmes.

2. More accuracy in determining effect and no-effect levels, both for short- and long-term exposures.

3. Consequent greater accuracy in predicting harmful effects and in some cases the suppression of harmful syndromes (e.g. quenching of the sensitizing potential of certain aldehydes[3]).

4. The elimination of pain and discomfort in animal and human studies.

5. The development of more sensitive epidemiology techniques.

6. All the above to be conducted on an acceptable cost/benefit basis.

The strategies we could employ are:

(i) The development of more accessible data banks and publishing and inclusion in data banks of negative data.

(ii) The replacement of maximization procedures involving pain and discomfort (e.g. Draize eye test, skin irritation tests progressed to corrosion, full LD-50 studies).

(iii) The development of alternative techniques such as:
    (a) more sophisticated tissue culture studies,
    (b) progress of in vitro mutagenicity and teratology studies,
    (c) development of in vitro sensitization studies,
    (d) progress in quantitative structure/activity relationship studies (QSARs).

(iv) The correlation of predictive and human diagnostic tests with clinical data (e.g. of positive skin patch and prick tests with human diseases such as dermatitis and asthma).

(v)   Improvement in correlation of animal tests with human experience.

(vi)   The establishment of an acceptable system for adverse reaction reporting.

(vii) The evaluation of cost/benefit by more sophisticated techniques than hitherto - leading to a rational approach to reasonable risk exposure.

Reasonable hazard awareness is an essential prerequisite to the initiation of a rational health and safety programme, whether this be by industry self-regulation or by decree of an enforcing authority. The hazard should then be carefully evaluated and quantified from existing data. The data studies will take several forms:

1.   Known toxicity data (animal and human).

2.   Extrapolation of animal data to man.

3.   Known human effects from manufacture or use of the material.

Subsequent testing should aim at remedying omissions in these data, but only if such tests provide meaningful data applicable to man or other species to be protected.
      Final effectual implementation of the health and safety programme demands close liaison between those generating the data, those who apply the programme and those who monitor for its success or failure as evidenced by any harmful sequelae.   It should be clear that this involves not only toxicologists, but also engineers, chemists, physicists, safety specialists, nurses and physicians, the latter adequately trained in occupational and environmental medicine.   The involvement of the physician is essential, for apart from his interest in matters biological and pharmacological, we depend on him for diagnosis when our system has failed, and for his opinion on the effects of potentially toxic agents on the unfit workmen as well as the fit, and are any of us without fault or defect?
      The days of "cook-book" toxicology, with its reliance on numbers (especially if statistically significant but of biological irrelevance) should be over.   Regrettably many legislative bodies concentrate more and more on such practices in the belief that a quantified experiment must be meaningful.   It is time we appreciated that a number or pass/failure code is only meaningful if it can be reliably repeated with the same results and if the result can be accurately and intelligently extrapolated to the question under consideration.
      It is true that Galileo said "Measure what you can measure, count what you can count - if there is no measurement, invent one"; since when scientists have often incorrectly assumed that unless a parameter can be measured it is not scientifically acceptable.

Even when measurement is practicable, it may be inaccurate - all measurements have a degree of potential error and this should be clearly defined and stated. Such determinations in biological studies are more variable than in physicochemical measurements of which Galileo was speaking.

The "OECD Guidelines for Testing of Chemicals"[1] refer to the use of the numerical value of the median lethal dose (LD-50) as widely used in toxicity classification systems, but point out that it should "not be regarded as an absolute number identifying the toxicity of a chemical substance". Nevertheless many do use it for just that purpose, and no official advice has yet been given in classification legislation on how to deal with varying results in multiple studies. The best advice is to make an informed judgement and the term "judgemental toxicology" is likely to be heard much more in the future.

"Cook-book" programmes would be justifiable if they had been shown to decrease the risks to human health and safety, but in many cases the evidence for this is meagre. In retrospect one may think of a test which would have been useful (e.g. as in the assessment of the toxicity of thalidomide), but it is impossible to carry out all tests on every chemical; it should not need stating that there are just not enough laboratories, animals or toxicologists to carry out more than a fraction of such full testing programmes. We should concentrate on those likely to lead to data of biological significance (e.g. determination of absorption, target organs and the pathology of lesions produced). Our ultimate criterion of acceptability of risk should be that we would be prepared for those nearest and dearest to us to be exposed to the chemical under consideration and in the manner proposed.

While numerical classifications seem to be generally acceptable to the community, the concept of the judgemental process is frequently looked upon with distrust, although lip-service is paid to it in some regulatory situations. Reasoned judgements or informed opinions appear to some to hint at an unjustified "superior" or even biased opinion - and yet it is often a most essential stage of any decision-making process in respect of health and safety programmes.

Perhaps the scientist has been too self-assured in the past and he has been too anxious to give a definitive opinion without justification of possible degree of error. In other cases inadequate training or inability to update basic experience may be to blame. Certainly training in toxicology is often inadequate, and the linking of biochemistry, animal toxicology and medical science deficient. The test data and epidemiological experience must be correlated with normal and abnormal exposure to normal (fit) and abnormal (unfit) humans. We must not be guilty, as Dostoyevsky wrote - "They have analysed the parts and overlooked the whole and indeed their blindness is marvellous." We must not only train others in toxicology and associated sciences but "pace each other along the paths of excellence".

The extrapolation of animal test data to man often requires comparative kinetic and metabolic studies in both animal and man if one is to form a reasonable judgement. One only has to study the question of carcinogenicity of coumarin - does it exist in animals to a significant extent and if so is it referable to man? Other studies, such as some on skin or eye irritation, are more easily inter-relatable. Freeburg and co-workers have described such correlation for household products[4].

The determination of effect/no-effect levels and their theoretical determination for man depends upon a judgement of the applicability of the available animal data to man. Where direct studies on man are practicable without undue harm then these are desirable. An example of such studies might include those for evaluation of possible visual effects of chemicals. With access to more sophisticated equipment, and especially of analytical techniques, determination of the metabolism and fate of very small doses of chemicals in man is now more practicable. Radiotracers can be used at detectable acceptable levels in many experiments where determination of absorption, metabolism or target organ is important.

The use of "alternative techniques" in place of animal studies is very much in the minds of all toxicologists[5]. However, so far there is no way in which a complete evaluation programme can be satisfactorily effected without some recourse to animal studies. The use of anything other than completely necessary tests is to be deprecated and in vivo studies may replace some tests and minimize others. They may well be more efficient in some instances, especially in the investigative field. Until we find more fully acceptable in vitro tests, recourse to standard protocols will of necessity continue, but some tests in standard legislative protocols could well be discontinued now. A full LD-50 is rarely, if ever, necessary and gives singularly little useful data. Many alternative techniques for the study of acute toxicity have been suggested and pressure should be brought on legislative and other administrative bodies to discontinue such requirements, convenient as they may be for purposes of classification. Zbinden and Flury-Roversi have discussed the significance of the LD-50 test for the toxicological evaluation of chemical substances[6], and Chanter and Heywood have discussed some considerations of precision[7].

The same applies to most standard rabbit eye tests. These could easily be modified to give as much or more data while producing only minimal changes in the eye (i.e. by establishing a minimal effect dose). In vitro studies already give valuable data to estimate a rank order of eye irritancy between chemicals of similar structure, and this could be utilized in designing eye test protocols.

The study of structure/activity is receiving increasing support and while it cannot be relied upon for completely definitive answers, with the increased recording and dissemination of data, it is frequently possible to anticipate toxic sequelae and thereby minimize testing in some cases. The availability of computer modelling has facilitated highly sophisticated studies of many toxicity problems. Craig[8] has indicated that such modelling for estimation of the LD-50 from a large data base may be more accurate than experimental tests on only three or four animals at three or four doses. He mentions the considerable variation in experimental toxicity data, referred to earlier in this paper, due to many factors enumerated by Zbinden and Flury-Roversi[6]. Weir, Simmons and Fan[9] have described a method for abstracting dose-response information from published studies for use in quantitative structure/activity relationships (QSARs). The ability to study skin penetration by mathematical modelling has proved useful in the drug industry and could with advantage be used more frequently in the study of industrial chemicals.

Factors to consider in the strategy for design of a testing programme might therefore include:

1. Degree of reassurance required.
2. Time schedule.
3. Cost.
4. A secondary strategy if any results are found to be unacceptable.

These various factors can with advantage be considered in a "critical path" analysis.

The minimal and "reasonably optimal" degree of reassurance required will involve consideration of legal requirements, industrial self-regulatory standards and the possible volume of various modes of use anticipated, immediately and over specific time frames. Such considerations will determine the types of test required and in some situations the detailed protocols. For example, in the EEC, the types of test required for a new chemical are defined according to volume produced and mode of use.

The time available will determine whether the tests have to be conducted concurrently or sequentially. The advantage of the latter is that the expense of a total programme can be reduced by modifications or cancellation of an original tentative programme in the event of a significant untoward result in one test. An example might be an unexpected high level of toxicity in an acute oral toxicity range-finding test. This might render the chemical unsuitable for use and thereby preclude the total testing programme envisaged.

Cost may dictate the practicability of a more extensive testing programme and "worst possible case" estimates should be prepared to allow for unforeseen adverse effects. The latter would lead to a secondary strategy which might be cessation of further studies or the pursuit of further tests to elucidate areas of doubt. An example would be the study of dermal penetration, metabolic pathways and kinetics when there is a marked apparent discrepancy between oral and dermal toxicity studies.

However, it is imperative that all concerned in the safety evaluation programme appreciate that further testing may not of itself solve such problems. Such tests may confirm that the problem exists; the overall strategy for any testing programme must always take account of the possibility of unacceptability of the product for its intended use and any consequent action thereby necessitated. The use of "critical path" analysis techniques for toxicity testing, marketing and sales programmes in the early stages of development of a chemical may save significantly, both in time and total costs incurred.

A self-critical approach to testing programmes is highly desirable and the same applies to legislation programmes. A vast

114

amount of health and safety legislation has been introduced in the past few years. This should be evaluated to assess whether it has had the desired results and whether any improvement in health and safety can be properly ascribed to such legislation or whether, if such improvement is demonstrated, it is due to other factors. In short there should be constant audit of the effectiveness of such legislation. If future legislative and other control programmes are to be developed along effective but economic lines, a decision-tree approach for the estimation of toxic hazards can be used to prioritize essential testing[10].

There will be a need for more fully trained specialists of high calibre, especially of toxicologists. The support of training programmes in health and safety services, especially toxicology and environmental medicine, should be considered of the highest priority if the anticipated benefits of current and prospective legislation are to be achieved.

In conclusion, one should refer to data quality assurance. The principles of good laboratory practice (GLP), as enunciated by several authorities, have done much to raise standards and consequently the reliability of reports. Noel[11] has discussed quality assurance in respect to the use of laboratory animals. By a rigid adherence to the best practices and a constant endeavour to render our work and conclusions more meaningful, we can continue to pace each other along those desirable paths of excellence.

REFERENCES

1. OECD (19) Guidelines for testing of chemicals. (Paris: OECD)
2. Fed Reg (1984). 49, 25082
3. Opdyke, DLJ (1976). Inhibition of sensitization reactions induced by certain aldehydes. Fd Cosmet Toxicol, 14, 197-8
4. Freeburg, FE, Griffiths, JF, Bruce, RD and Bay, PHS (1984). Correlation of animal test methods with human experience for household products. J Toxicol Cut Ocular Toxicol, 1, 53-64
5. Balls, M, Riddell, RJ and Worden, AN (eds) (1983). Animals and Alternatives in Toxicity Testing. (London: Academic Press)
6. Zbinden, G and Flury-Roversi, M (1981). Arch Toxicol, 47, 77-99
7. Chanter, DO and Heywood, R (1982). The LD-50 test: some considerations of precision. Toxicol Lett, 10, 303-7
8. Craig, PN (1983). Mathematical models for toxicity evaluations. Ann Rep Med Chem, 18, 303-6
9. Weir, BR, Simmons, WS, Fan, AM, Livingston, DL, Tesche, NS and Walton, AH (1981). Development of a format for abstracting dose-response information from published studies for use in quantitative structure-activity relationships (QSARs). J Chem Inf Comput Sci, 21, 14-18
10. Cramer, GM, Ford, RA and Hall, RL (1978). Estimation of toxic hazard - a decision-tree approach. Fed Cosmet Toxicol, 6, 255

11. Noel, PRB (1982). Toxicity testing, hazard assessment and data quality assurance in respect to use of laboratory animals. In Bartosek, I (ed.) Toxicology Research (New York: Raven Press)

9

Evaluating the Hazards of Pesticides

G. J. TURNBULL

INTRODUCTION

Pesticides provide important benefits in agriculture and public health[1,2] and the balance of evidence shows that these chemicals are not producing an epidemic of poisoning[1,3-6]. However, some aspects of present hazard evaluation procedures can be criticized.

This chapter summarizes the way pesticides are evaluated for hazard to man and to the environment, and discusses those aspects where change either is needed or is inevitable.

Pesticide is an omnibus term for chemicals used in agriculture, horticulture and public health programmes to control predatory forms of life. It indicates a function in one of the following categories[6]:

1. Insecticides, aphicides, miticides, nematocides, etc., directed against invertebrates which feed on crops, stored foods, farm or domestic animals, or people.

2. Fungicides to control, for example, the growth of mildew on plants, or fungi in stored foods.

3. Herbicides (weed killers) to control the growth of unwanted plants.

4. Plant growth regulators, for example, to limit the height of cereals.

5. Rodenticides to poison rats, mice and sometimes other vertebrates.

6. Protective agents for building materials.

For a very long time biologically active chemicals have been used to combat pests. The early attempts sometimes involved substances which were toxic to man, such as nicotine, arsenic, strychnine and phenol. In the past 40 years innovation in the chemical industry has produced a variety of pesticides which have been increasingly selective in their biological effects[7]. The history of pesticides shows that the benefits have been obtained as problems have been resolved. The organochlorine insecticides were highly beneficial in agriculture, and in public health their use saved many lives, for example in malaria control programmes[1,2]. Biological persistence is a characteristic of this group and their use has declined as alternatives were invented. Organophosphorus compounds succeeded them in widespread use but the anticholinesterase properties of these compounds (and also the carbamate insecticides developed more recently) present a potential acute hazard to people involved in pesticide application. Over-exposure has resulted in cases of poisoning and some fatalities[8,9]. Some herbicides also were rather toxic; for example, dinitro-ortho-cresol produced occasional cases of poisoning and some deaths[8,9]. During transport of pesticides there have been some accidents which caused contamination of food, particularly flour, and outbreaks of acute poisoning[9,10].

To control the increasing use of pesticides many developed countries devised voluntary or statutory schemes regulating the packing, labelling and use of such chemicals[11]. There is now a variety of efficacious pesticides covering the various categories of pesticide use and diverse chemical families are represented. The regulations which apply to pesticides are comprehensive and, although the details differ between countries[11], their purpose is simple. First, there are regulations which protect people occupationally exposed to the pesticides they are handling, wherever they are working. Second, the officially approved uses of pesticides specify the crops and limit the time of application in the growing season (and the frequency of application) in order to ensure that pesticide residues in human or animal food or the environment do not reach levels which may cause harm[10]. Third, there are requirements to provide information on the potential hazards of the product during transport, storage and use, and this is done by product labels and packaging inserts giving advice and cautionary statements. Moreover the type of container is controlled in many national schemes. National authorities require information from the manufacturer and perform an independent safety evaluation before permitting any sale of a new pesticide. The information for these premarketing evaluations is extensive, and it may be re-examined if sales continue over the years.

Chemicals with pesticidal activity are seldom used without the addition of carriers, solvent, wetting agents or diluent. These so-called inert ingredients in the commercial formulation (i.e. the product) may modify the acute toxicity of the pesticide, sometimes significantly. The physical form of the product often is a liquid in which the pesticide active ingredient is dissolved or is present as an emulsion or a suspension. Generally such liquid formulations are dispersed in water prior to application, as are wettable powder formulations. Powders containing a small proportion of pesticide active ingredient are used where a dry, penetrating treatment is needed while granules provide a way of releasing the pesticide at the target in the soil. Pesticides used in the home and garden, including aerosol insecticides, are dilute formulations, providing an additional margin of safety.

There is only limited standardization of the equipment used to apply pesticides. The rate of application of the pesticides to the crop, livestock or buildings involved, and the physical nature of the formulation, determine the design of the equipment. Depending on how the application equipment is designed and used, the exposure to pesticides which people receive may be extremely low or significantly large[12].

PESTICIDE EXPOSURE AND SAFETY

Evaluations are carried out independently by the pesticide manufacturer and the national regulatory authorities with the objective of ensuring a reasonable expectation of minimal adverse effects from the recommended uses (or indeed from the misuses which might reasonably be predicted). In summary, the benefits must outweigh the risks. However, some authorities adopt procedures in the administration of their regulations consistent with a policy of requiring absolute freedom from adverse effects, including responses of an extremely hypothetical nature. There is therefore a distinction between safety studies and so-called regulatory toxicology.

Even very toxic chemicals can be used effectively and safely provided the exposure of people (and the contamination of the environment) is reduced in proportion, according to the hazard. Information on exposure is as important as information on the toxicity of the pesticide[4,13,14]. Depending on the intended use of the pesticide and its toxicity (qualitative and quantitative) a variety of procedures and precautions are required by authorities, such as wearing protective gloves, which can control the exposure[14].

The toxic properties of a material, however, are immutable. The problem is to identify the properties, quantify them in terms of a dose-response relationship, and define the relevance of the findings to man (or other target species in the environment). The so-called no-effect level is derived from the dose-response information, i.e. the dose level which evokes no observable adverse response in the target organism.

The state of the art for safety testing is to employ surrogate test systems (often laboratory animals) to study acute and chronic poisoning. Unless there is evidence to the contrary, it is assumed that, qualitatively, man is as susceptible as the laboratory animals. Quantitatively, for the assessment of hazard, it is frequently assumed that man is a hundred-fold more susceptible than laboratory animals, thereby introducing a safety factor of this magnitude in risk calculations.

Occupational exposure to pesticides is, with few exceptions, predominantly by skin contact[4,12] while the general population may be exposed to pesticides or their metabolites at low levels by ingestion of residues in food[1,10]. Only rarely is there potential inhalation of pesticide, for example during fumigation of buildings[4,12]. There is extensive published information on occupational exposure to pesticides[12] and for each pesticide used on food crops extensive information is obtained at an early stage on residue levels in foodstuffs and the environment. To simulate likely human exposure to pesticides the toxicity studies are performed using a variety of routes and durations of exposure.

TOXICITY TESTING

Early in the programme of safety studies the identity and physicochemical properties of the active ingredient, and details of any impurities in the manufactured material, are defined so that representative material is used in the toxicity and environmental studies[11].

Acute toxicity

Acute toxicity by the oral and dermal route, and irritancy to the skin and eye, are studied both for the pesticidal active ingredient and the formulation on sale. The sensitizing potential of the active ingredient is also investigated. Inhalational toxicity of the active ingredient is studied unless, for example, it is a highly viscous liquid at room temperature. Commonly regulatory authorities also require inhalation toxicity data on the (undiluted) formulation even if there is no opportunity for generating particles of respirable size in the breathing zone of farm or public health workers. This demand reflects an unwarranted preoccupation with inhalational exposure, perhaps due to the smell many pesticides create locally during application, and a need to identify a hazard category for labelling purposes. Irritancy to the skin or eye, or significant acute toxicity by any route, confers an obligation to label the containers and product information with warning signs and symbols, for the protection of people during transport, storage, distribution and use.

It is the need to have distinct categories for hazard labelling which obliges authorities to request LD-50 and LC-50 values. These numerical data are of limited value. The most important information is the nature, severity and time course of symptoms of acute poisoning. This, together with evidence of a dose-response relationship, can lead to recommendations for the diagnosis and treatment of acute poisoning.

Repeated dose and long-term studies

Only if there is the likelihood of recurrent gross skin contamination of workers, or if acute irritancy studies suggest a problem, are repeated dermal exposure studies undertaken with the formulation. The active ingredient per se is invariably subjected to repeated dose and long-term toxicity studies. Typically the initial requirement is for rat and dog 90-day toxicity studies by the oral route. The chemical is usually fed in the diet at constant concentration levels to different groups of animals. This is intended to imitate the human exposure presented by residues in crops and should also demonstrate a no-effect level. There will generally be a further requirement for chronic oral route data obtained in a 2-

year rat, an 18-month or 2-year mouse study and a multi-generation rat study. The effects of chronic exposure in a non-rodent species will be investigated in a 6- or 12-month dog study. The need for the chronic studies is generally linked to an intended use on human food crops where a finite residue is anticipated.

Each of these studies must span a range of doses from the clearly toxic to the (non-toxic) no-effect level. The problem is to characterize, in meaningful terms, toxicity at high dose levels and at the border of the no-effect level[13,14]. Comprehensive haematology, clinical chemistry and urine analysis studies are per-formed repeatedly in all multi-dose studies with the exception of reproduction studies such as the multi-generation rat study. At termination all animals in each type of study are examined for gross changes and for microscopic lesions by extensive histopathol-ogy. The weights of selected organs also are examined.

In order to study the effects of maternal exposure on the developing fetus, teratology studies in rat and rabbit are required. Impairment of fertility or general reproductive perfor-mance in the multi-generation studies, which comprises a minimum of two successive generations dosed continuously, may lead to fur-ther studies to characterize the effect.

Special studies may be required, depending on the findings in the above studies; for example, neurotoxicity investigations with cholinesterase-inhibiting organophosphorus compounds.

Detailed information also is required on the metabolism of the active ingredient in the rat and commonly also the dog. A metabo-lite which appears in plants but is not found in animals will be synthesized and subject to 90-day rat and dog toxicity tests.

Mutagenicity testing

Mutagenicity test data usually have to be provided on the pesticide active ingredient. The requirement may be limited to an Ames test; alternately a battery of up to five tests may be demanded, e.g. for Italy. As a general rule, however, the following data are adequate for regulatory purposes[13,15-17]:

1. A gene mutation study in a bacterial system (e.g. Ames test).

2. A chromosome damage assay in mammalian cells (e.g. metaphase chromosome analysis of cultured human lymphocytes).

3. A test for other genotoxic effects (e.g. gene mutation in mammalian cells, DNA damage or repair in mammalian cells, numerical chromosomal aberrations, mammalian cell transforma-tion, target organ/gonad germ cell damage).

Mutagenicity testing is one of the problem areas for both the manufacturers and authorities[17,18]. There is no difficulty in detecting genotoxic activity and, in fact, there are too many dif-ferent assays[19]. The US EPA identifies about 40 options for mutagenicity testing[16], few of which are validated[20]. There are no standardized protocols for many of the tests and so the value of data from such assays is questionable. The mouse lymphoma L5178Y TK+/- system illustrates the dilemma. From a theoretical standpoint such mammalian cell gene mutation data should be useful if a chemical is to be judged for potential human genotoxic· hazard. Unfortunately, artefactual results can be produced by, for example, altered pH or osmolarity, and so far there are no agreed criteria for a positive response in this system. Experience has shown that a positive (unfavourable) response is obtained with a large proportion of compounds of unknown carcinogenicity which otherwise appear not to be genotoxic[21]. The interpretation of such mutagenicity data presents a major problem, particularly with respect to carcinogenicity.

WILDLIFE AND ENVIRONMENT STUDIES

The potential environmental problems associated with the use of pesticides is the subject of frequent enquiry. There is widespread awareness of, for example, DDT transfer through food chains and its persistence in the environment[1,2]. Extensive information on the environmental fate of pesticides is now generated by manufacturers, and reviewed by the authorities prior to marketing[11,22]. Breakdown of the pesticide in crops, soil and water is studied both quantitatively and qualitatively, and effects on fish, aquatic invertebrates and soil organisms are assessed. Toxicity to birds and beneficial insects is investigated in the laboratory if the intended agricultural use of the pesticide seems likely to expose these species in the field. In addition to environmental safety studies the authorities in a number of countries insist that the manufacturers must submit data to show that the product is efficacious. In some countries, such as Germany and Holland, efficacy trials are also carried out by government establishments[11].

RESIDUES

Residues data are required by the regulatory authorities to assess, in conjunction with the toxicological data, any hazard to consumers from the proposed use of the pesticide, and also to define any risk to workers handling the treated crops[1,10,11]. The amount and nature of the residues and the rate of decline are indentified in the relevant crops[23-25]. When poultry or livestock are exposed to pesticides, either by consumption of treated foodstuffs or, for example, by external treatment for ectoparasite control, then residue levels in meat, milk or eggs are measured. Despite considerable investigation there is no consistent evidence of adverse health effects in man due to pesticide residues which arise in foodstuffs from typical agricultural practice[9,10].

HEALTH EFFECTS OF PESTICIDES

Past performance is not always a reliable guide to the future. In the case of pesticide safety, the record of occupational and non-occupational illness and deaths provides a strong indication of the future trends. The information on adverse health effects from developed countries and the developing countries have recently been reviewed[1,3-5,26]. The safety record of pesticides generally is good.

Postmarketing surveillance of pesticide safety involves the manufacturer, the regulatory authorities which control pesticides in the various countries, and regional poisoning and control centres. The manufacturer is well placed to obtain and collect information on accidents or poisonings involving its products. Some companies are particularly diligent in this form of product stewardship but there is no statutory obligation to collect or analyse such information. In the developed countries, cases of alleged poisoning by pesticides often are formally investigated by a government-appointed body[4]. While there has been concern that such investigations suffer from a degree of under-reporting it is felt that all serious and fatal cases in developed countries are well documented. However, some of the more minor cases of, for example, skin irritation may go unreported[4]. In contrast, the developing countries have few means of gathering reliable information and cases seldom are formally recorded or investigated[26].

FUTURE NEEDS

Pesticide hazard evaluation procedures have proved very effective, but nonetheless some changes are necessary. In the course of protecting people, and the environment, from potentially hazardous pesticides government authorities have to implement decisions which are politically unpopular, for example to groups such as Friends of the Earth. Length reviews, bureaucratic delay and unending demand for more safety studies are features of the official decision-making process. Scientists performing the safety studies find that reasonable progress is impeded by regulations which mingle empericism, established scientific fact, unverified scientific theory and political expediency. The costs of unnecessary studies and added administration have to be passed on to the farmers and to agencies funding public health or amenity programmes, and so food production and health suffer, particularly in the developing and least-developed countries. In the developed countries, which enjoy a high standard of living, there is public concern for safety and fears of lingering harm to people and the environment. There can be no doubt that the regulations controlling pesticides will be refined in response to these various, sometimes conflicting, pressures. Further rules and controls seem inevitable but they may not be necessary.

Health information

While it is helpful to understand the scientific basis for safety measures it is not essential; sometimes understanding the science comes after the problem was solved. For example the earlier problems of over-exposure to pesticides and occupational poisoning by, for example, parathion and DNOC, have been solved. There are less hazardous, more efficacious and convenient products and protective procedures and precautions have been refined[1]. However, more could be done to protect the innocent victims of malpractice such as the transfer of pesticide from the original labelled container to unlabelled domestic bottles kept in the home[1,14]. The need is to convey experience and know-how to the developing countries, and to obtain reliable information on occupational and public health from those countries[1,3,14]. Theoretical models of pesticide poisoning[5] are no substitute for the facts[3]. Some form of monitoring, or audit for poisoning by pesticides in selected developing countries, would be valuable provided the sovereignty of governments was not infringed. The problem lies in obtaining reliable information.

Pesticide regulation

Regulation of pesticides is an arena where the pragmatists confront the purists who seek absolute assurance that products are not harmful. The quest for infallibility has proliferated test requirements and led to the specification of more and more studies in greater and greater detail[1]. The United States EPA is in the forefront of this movement, but the trend is widespread.

Protocols for test methods which are routinely specified by authorities continue to be refined but there is a need for regulatory authorities to acknowledge the inherent fallacies in detailed guidelines. The imposition of guidelines as bureaucratic rules rather than as pointers towards genuine understanding hinder hazard evaluations. New assay procedures must be introduced but, unlike some tests in current guidelines, the new assays must have been adequately shown to be reproducible, reliable and practicable in laboratories world-wide. The criteria for adverse or favourable findings in new assays need to be decided before new assays are used in decision-making processes, not afterwards, as is presently the case in some countries. The mouse lymphoma mutagenicity assay described earlier illustrates the point. The United States EPA considers the assay a suitable basis for decision-making[13,27] despite its acknowledged imprecision. The EPA approach to mutagenicity risk assessment makes no provision for the uncertainties inherent in many of the mutagenicity assays[27] and, by requiring a battery of tests, reduces the likelihood that any new pesticide will have completely favourable safety data. It has been suggested that the current range of mutagenicity testing guidelines is unnecessarily complex and as such may actually be damaging industry without a commensurate advantage to human health[19]. The immediate need is to make thoughtful use of two, and a maximum of three, assays of proven

124

reliability and established relevance to man[18-21,28]. These comments on the introduction of new assays are particularly relevant at a time when considerable efforts are being made to develop new test methods with the intention of reducing the numbers of animals used by laboratories in the course of safety testing of chemicals.

Improved test methods

Even when test methods have been widely used there remains scope for improvement in the choice of parameters to be measured, but progress appears to be slow. In part this can be attributed to the stultifying effect of detailed test guidelines.

For example, the clinical biochemists can now measure up to 20 parameters on 200 µl or less of plasma. Which parameters are useful diagnostic indicators and are directly relevant to man? In the rat and dog, gamma-glutamyl transpeptidase plasma levels are lower than in man and not generally useful as indicators of tissue damage, although these parameters are recommended in the OECD guidelines[29]. Measurement of lactate dehydrogenase (LDH) levels assists in the diagnosis of coronary heart failure in man, and was in the guidelines the EPA originally proposed[30]. However, this parameter loses its significance in animal toxicity studies which use a maximum tolerated dose since a variety of tissues probably affect the LDH plasma levels in laboratory animals; furthermore some species and strain differences are likely. Ornithine decarboxylase assays are included in the OECD guidelines[29], referred to by some authorities, but the value of this parameter in clinical diagnosis in laboratory animals is largely unproven. Conversely, glutamate dehydrogenase and ornithine carbamoyltransferase appear to be useful markers for liver tissue damage in laboratory animals although these parameters are not requested by authorities and are not routine screening parameters in human studies.

There is considerable pressure on laboratories to comply with protocols in official guidelines, in every detail. Rejection of a study by an authority is the ultimate sanction and can be a very major commercial penalty. Few laboratories would omit to fast the rats and dogs in subchronic and chronic studies for blood glucose measurement, as required by the present EPA guidelines[16], despite the indications that the fasting period is a gratuitous procedure. It provides minimal additional clinical information but does cause some additional stress. The clinical chemistry parameters in animal toxicity studies need to be refined so that meaningful data are recognized by the regulatory authorities.

Modern haematology analyses combine cellular counting with computation of cell volume, size, and size distribution skewness. The diagnostic potential of changes in cell size distribution has yet to be assessed although the method is convenient and precise. Cell size is a sensitive indicator of effects on red blood cell production and destruction, and this parameter is likely to contribute to the design of future toxicity studies.

THE FUTURE OF PREDICTIVE SAFETY EVALUATION

Extrapolation to man

The future of predictive safety evaluations of pesticides lies in deciding more precisely the relevance to man and his environment of certain toxic changes seen only in model systems. In that way the acceptability of the predicted margins of safety can be examined more clearly and more openly.

When the many reports on safety studies on a pesticide are examined during a hazard evaluation there is no single calculation, or checklist, which allows a reliable prediction of the toxic hazard resulting from excessive exposure, for example during an accident or misuse of a product. An element of judgement is required[2,10,13] and the weight given to individual pieces of information should reflect the relevance of that information to man. However, the scientific foundation for this discretionary aspect in the interpretation of toxicity data is far from complete. Regulatory authorities are forced, therefore, to adopt somewhat arbitrary policies for data interpretation[31]. The Delaney Clause is an important example.

In the USA the so-called Delaney Clause in the food laws prohibits the use of a pesticide or chemical if it is found to induce cancer when determined by an appropriate test[32]. A problem to be resolved is what test is deemed appropriate[31]. Crucial to the interpretation of test data is the question of there being either a threshold dose for certain carcinogenic effects in animals or a carcinogenic hazard (in theory) from a small dose or even a single molecule[2,33-36]. Mrak[2] and others[18] have concluded that so far neither possibility had been proved. Meanwhile a number of authorities assume that there can be no threshold dose for carcinogens and go so far as to calculate hypothetical risks to man due to the use of certain pesticides and food additives. There are several mathematical models which are said to estimate the risk to man of low-level exposure to chemical carcinogens from animal tumour data[13,17,33-39]. None of the models can actually be based on the biological processes in operation until the carcinogenic process is better understood[28,32,36,40]. The data from animal experiments of a realistic size do not allow the rejection, on statistical grounds, of the hypothesis that the carcinogenic reponse to a chemical is positive even at very low dosage levels[33,35,38]. Tolerance distribution models assume that there is a tolerance level, which differs between individuals, so there is not a single threshold for a population, while stochastic models assume that a carcinogenic response reflects the probability of one or more "chemical hits" on the system[35,38]. If the upper confidence limits from such models are used to calculate notional human risk then even the smallest exposure involves a putative risk of cancer[37,38]. The US EPA is prominent in the use of such estimates in the decision process for pesticide registration, but the apparent precision is an illusion based upon a flawed approach.

Calculations of human cancer risk from chemicals by statistical models which are solely founded on arbitrary assumptions[35] or hypotheses in biology, are a negation of science in the majority of cases. An hypothesis which cannot be tested by experimentation is not a scientific hypothesis[34], although it may be fashionable dogma[35]. The hypothesis that there is no no-effect level for carcinogen exposure is an example of a negative hypothesis that cannot be confirmed or refuted[33], and it is having a stultifying, rather than a stimulating, effect on the quality of safety evaluations. In fact the data in support of a no-threshold chemical induction of tumours in man are sparse and inconclusive[33]. However, the alternative hypothesis, postulating threshold dose levels for carcinogens, is supported by some published experimental evidence[33,34] and a significant amount of unpublished data.

Purchase[41] described the assumptions being made in such calculation of a putative human cancer risk as unreasonable and considered the dispersion of the resulting human risk estimates to indicate lack of precision and reliability. There is general confidence in the ability of the animal bioassay to detect potential human carcinogens. However, attempts to quantify human risk on the basis of such studies by means of mathematical models is subject to very considerable uncertainty[33,36,40,42-45]. The ingenuity involved in the various models has to be admired, but the accuracy of ultraconservative calculations is discredited. Consider the case of the fumigant ethylene dibromide. The calculated human risk from the actual level of human exposure was substantial, but the observed mortality indicated no occupational increase in risk[45]. Evidently the assumptions made in the model led to an exaggeration of the calculated risk. Such calculations suggest that there is a broadly similar degree of human risk from low-level exposure to aflatoxin, vinyl chloride or dimethylnitrosamine as from saccharin, ethylene dibromide, DDT, dieldrin or formaldehyde[34,35,38,39,41,44-46]. The accuracy of the calculations is inadequate and the apparent precision offered by alternative models serves only to confuse the hazard assessment. The effective dose to the target organ, rather than the administered dose given to the animal, is important in estimating the response to low-level exposure. Exposing people to potent genotoxic carcinogens obviously is more hazardous than equal exposure to non-mutagenic chemicals which produce only tumours of doubtful relevance to man in chronically poisoned animals.

As a general rule there is ample published information to show that such human risk calculations have no relevance to, and so should not be employed in, the following cases:

1. Chemically induced tumours were present only in animals suffering an alteration in the physiological or endocrine status due to dosages clearly above the maximum tolerated dose. Hormone-dependent tumours in chronically poisoned rodents usually are of very doubtful relevance to man.

2. The chemical-induced tumours due to local effects in the target tissue and the local effects either do not, or cannot, occur in man. For example, liver tumours in mice, and possibly also rats, are not necessarily indicators of a carcinogenic hazard to man[18,47]. Likewise, chronic gross irritation of the upper respiratory tract leading to local tumour

formation in the rat does not prove that a chemical is an occupational cancer hazard since people will not tolerate persistent severe respiratory tract irritation.

Clearly there is a need to evaluate chemicals on a case-by-case
basis[13,17,18,28,30,31,43,44,48], but there is a great need to
question the relevance to man of certain findings, and to refine
the procedures used in toxicity tests[13,17,18,36].

Spurious and uninterpretable findings in chronic studies do
not promote safety and need to be avoided. There needs to be
more emphasis on the interpretation of findings in the investigations used to establish dose levels for the chronic studies. Even
in mice, where clinical chemistry and haematology parameters are
not customary in chronic studies (except for Japan), there should
be a comprehensive examination of these parameters in the
preparatory tests to establish dose levels for the chronic study.
Measurement of plasma levels of several hormones can now be made
in rodents, and the implications of any treatment-related changes
need to be considered before the start of the chronic studies and
not left to the end when tumours have been found. Likewise, if
there is any indication of chemically induced liver enlargement in
rodents then comprehensive studies of drug-metabolizing enzyme
activity are essential. These should identify chemical induction of
cytochrome P-450 enzymes, including those associated with
peroxisome proliferation. As a general rule, a dose level which
chronically alters the metabolic, physiological or endocrine status
to a slight, but measurable, extent needs to be accepted as the
suitable highest dose level. Use of a maximum tolerated dose,
based solely on overt signs such as reduced body weight gain,
reduced water or food consumption or increased mortality, is
evidence of poor experimental design, although this method for setting dose levels is still officially advocated[13,18,49]. Such
changes may indicate ill-health, distress and suffering[50] and
there are ethical reasons as well as scientific arguments for avoiding dose levels which chronically induce such gross changes. The
same principle also applies to reproduction and teratology studies,
since overt poisoning of the dam will sometimes alter the incidence
of spontaneous fetal abnormalities. This can sometimes be attributed to a stress effect involving the dam, rather than a direct
effect on the fetus. However, it may be difficult to assuage a
suspicion of a teratogenic effect even though the true risk was
death of the mother rather than fetal abnormality.

COMMENT

There is a need for an holistic approach to the safety testing of
chemicals. Long-term experience in engineering and the physical
or chemical sciences has resulted in safety evaluation procedures
which involve examination both of the component parts or subsys-
tems and the complete unit. The ultimate test is performance under full load, or during use. Likewise to evaluate the safety of
chemicals there can be studies on model systems in vitro but these
do not, at present, show what will actually happen in the complete

organism. Properly designed experiments in laboratory animals effectively predict potential toxic hazards for man. However, epidemiological studies are the only way of showing that the predications for the safe use of chemicals are reliable, and that people have not been harmed by their exposure to the particular chemical[17,18].

The safety of people exposed to pesticides is now investigated in great detail, and there is no apparent gap in the premarketing screening of a new pesticide. In fact the need is to examine adverse findings in model systems rather more rigorously for their relevance to man. Not all findings in toxicity studies (including genotoxicity tests) can be extrapolated to man, and this needs to be more widely acknowledged. The protocols for some of the routine toxicity studies can be further refined and the means of dose level selection particularly needs to take advantage of the recent technical improvements in clinical chemistry and hormone assays in rodents.

Toxicity studies are performed primarily in order to investigate the safety of chemicals and so it is as well to remember that toxic chemicals have threatened man and animals since before recorded history. Many plants and a variety of insects and fungi produce toxic substances which effectively modify the local biological environment[32]. Ames[51] and others[1,32,52,53] have noted that plants in nature synthesize toxic chemicals in large amounts as a primary defence against bacterial, fungal and insect and other animal predators. The estimated human dietary intake of natural pesticides is likely to be several grams per day and probably at least 10,000 times higher than the dietary intake of man made pesticides[32,51]. Dietary intake of potent toxins such as aflatoxin can be between 0.25 and 3 μg person per day[32,39]. Some individuals consume considerably higher amounts and have an increased risk of liver cancer, as would be predicted from animal test data[39].

Many plants inhibit the growth of adjacent vegetation by means of chemicals released by volatilization, leaching from the stem and leaves or directly into the soil (allelopathy)[54,55] and there are insects which naturally secrete some highly toxic chemicals[54]. Oil from the neem tree (Azadirachta indica) may have some commercial potential as an insecticide in agriculture although it is, apparently, not completely non-toxic to mammals. Little information is available about the toxicology, and hence safety in use, of neem oil, or other natural plant toxins in food[51]. Aflatoxin is one of the relatively few examples of an intensively studied natural toxin in our food[32,39,52,53]. Both water and soil contain natural mutagens[56]. The food eaten by people, and laboratory animals, contains carcinogens and anticarcinogens, mutagens and various toxins[56,57] which contribute significantly to the incidence of so-called spontaneous tumours and degenerative pathological changes[51,57]. To view the possible hazards of pesticide residues in food in isolation from this natural background is misleading.

Given the chemically hostile nature of food and drinking water, the natural cellular biochemical repair processes and the operation of immunological surveillance in vivo, a threshold for carcinogenic effects of chemicals is more than a possibility[18,33]. A non-linear dose-response curve, involving thresholds for many toxic responses, is, on the weight of the evidence, a clear probability. The difficulty lies in marshalling the evidence to the satisfaction of regulatory authorities and deciding what safety margins should be applied with the various types of carcinogens, or other toxic substances, with widely differing potencies.

The future of safety evaluation of pesticides lies in establishing a firm scientific foundation so that the relevance to man of the various toxic changes can be decided[17,31]. Safety margins need to be defined more precisely, to reflect both the toxic properties and the benefits of the particular use[28]. Finally, the available information on human exposure could be exploited more fully and rationally. In summary, a review of the science involved in pesticide safety evaluations shows a number of aspects where progress is possible. Some changes are needed in these safety evaluations if the empiricism so far employed is to develop into a coherent, technically competent analysis of risk.

ACKNOWLEDGEMENTS

The advice from excellent colleagues, particulary Dr Marion Jackson, Kevin Rush and Dr David Foulkes, and the support of FBC Limited is gratefully acknowledged.

REFERENCES

1.   Buchel, KH (1984). Political economic and philosophical aspects of pesticide use for human welfare. Regul Toxicol Pharmacol, 4, 174-91

2.   Mrak, EM (1984). Pesticides: the good and the bad. Regul Toxicol Pharmacol, 4, 28-36

3.   Goulding, R (1983). Poisoning on the farm. J Soc Occup Med, 33, 60-5

4.   Bonsall, JL (1985). Pesticides and health in developed countries. In Turnbull, GJ (ed.) Occupational Hazards of Pesticide Use. pp. 51-66. (Basingstoke: Taylor and Francis)

5.   Copplestone, JF (1985). Pesticide exposure and health in developing countries. In Turnbull, GJ (ed.) Occupational Hazards of Pesticide Use. pp. 51-66. (Basingstoke: Taylor and Francis)

6.   Goulding, R (1985). Pesticide safety. In Turnbull, GJ (ed.) Occupational Hazards of Pesticide Use. pp. 1-12. (Basingstoke: Taylor and Francis)

7.   Corbett, JR, Wright, K and Baillie, AC (1984). The Biochemical Mode of Action of Pesticides. (London: Academic Press)

8.   Hearn, CED (1973). A review of agricultural pesticide incidents in man in England and Wales, 1952-71. Br J Indust Med, 30, 253-8

9.   Hayes, WJ (1982). Pesticides Studied in Man. (Baltimore:

Williams and Wilkins)
10. Turnbull, GJ (1984). Pesticide residues in food - a toxicological view. J Roy Soc Med, 77, 932-5
11. Thomas, B (1983). Pesticide Registration in the United Kingdom and Europe. Pesticide Residues, Ministry of Agriculture Fisheries and Food pp. 211-218. Ref. book 347. (London: HMSO)
12. Turnbull, GJ, Sanderson, DM and Crome, SJ (1985). Exposure to pesticides during application. In Turnbull, GJ (ed.) Occupational Hazards of Pesticide Use. pp. 35-49. (Basingstoke: Taylor and Francis)
13. EPA (1984). Proposed guidelines for carcinogen risk assessment. Fed Reg, 49, 46294-301
14. Turnbull, GJ (1985). Current trends and future needs. In Turnbull, GJ (ed.) Occupational Hazards of Pesticide Use. pp. 99-116. (Basingstoke: Taylor and Francis)
15. Committee on Mutagenicity of Chemicals in Food, Consumer Products and the Environment (1981). Guidelines for the Testing of Chemicals for Mutagenicity. DHSS Report on Health and Social Subjects No. 24. (London: HMSO)
16. EPA (1982). Pesticides Assessment Guidelines, Sub division F Hazard Evaluation Human and Domestic Animals. (Springfield: National Technical Information Service)
17. Interdisciplinary Panel on Carcinogenity (1984). Criteria for evidence of chemical carcinogenicity. Science, 225, 682-7
18. Jennings, JD (1985). Chemical Carcinogens; A Review of the Science and its Associated Principles, Part II: State of the Science. Office of Science and Technology Policy. Fed Reg, 10371-442 14 March
19. Ashby, J (1984). A logical approach to the detection of carcinogens and mutagens. In Critical Evaluation of Mutagenicity Tests. BGA Schriften 3/84, pp. 497-507. (Munich: MMV Medizin Verlag)
20. Garner, RC (1984). Comparison of results between whole animal studies and short-term tests for mutagenicity or carcinogenicity. In Critical Evaluation of Mutagenicity Tests. BGA Schriften 3/84, pp. 509-524. (Munich: MMV Medizin Verlag)
21. Shelby, MD and Stasiewicz, S (1984). Chemicals showing no evidence of carcinogenicity in long-term, two-species rodent studies: the need for short-term test data. Environ Mutagen, 6, 871-8
22. Thomas, B (1984). Pesticides and soils: a regulatory review. In Hance, RJ (ed.) Soils and Crop Protection Chemicals. pp. 15-23. British Crop Protection Council Monograph No. 27
23. Nicolson, RS (1984). Association of Public Analysts surveys of pesticide residues in Food, 1983. J Assoc Publ Analysts, 22, 51-7
24. MAFF (1982). Report of the Working Party on Pesticide Residues (1977-1981). Ministry of Agriculture Fisheries and Food. (London: HMSO)
25. GIFAP (1984). Pesticide Residues in Food. (Brussels: Groupment International des Associations Nationales De

Fabricants De Pesticides)

26. Jeyaratnam, J (1985). Health problems of pesticide usage in the Third World. Br J Indust Med, 42, 505-6

27. EPA (1984). Proposed guidelines for mutagenicity risk assessment. Fed Reg, 49, 46314-21

28. FAO/WHO (1984). Pesticide Residues in Food - Report of the Joint Meeting of the FAO Panel of Experts on Pesticide Residues in Food and the Environment and the WHO Expert Group on Pesticide Residues, Held in Geneva, 5 to 14 December 1983. FAO Plant Production and Protection Paper No. 56. (Rome: FAO)

29. OECD (1981). Guidelines for Testing of Chemicals. (Paris: OECD)

30. EPA (1978). Proposed Guidelines for Registering Pesticides, Subpart F. Fed Reg, 43, 37336-403

31. Goldstein, BD (1985). Risk assessment and risk management. Environ Toxicol Chem, 4, 1-2

32. Stitch, HF (ed.) (1982). Carcinogens and Mutagens in the Environment - Vol. I: Food Products. (Florida: CRC Press)

33. Maugh, TH (1978). Chemical carcinogens: how dangerous are low doses. Science, 202, 37-41

34. Clegg, DJ (1979). Animal reproduction and carcinogenicity studies in relation to human safety evaluation. Toxicol Occup Med, 4, 45-59

35. Guess, H, Crump, K and Peto, R (1977). Uncertainty estimates for low-dose rate extrapolations of animal carcinogenicity data. Cancer Res, 37, 3475-83

36. Krewski, D, Clayson, DB, Collins, B and Munro, IC (1982). Toxicological procedures for assessing the carcinogenic potential of agricultural chemicals. In Fleck, RA and Hollaender, A (eds) Genetic Toxicology, Basic Life Science Vol. 21. (New York: Plenum Press)

37. California Health and Welfare Agency (1982). Carcinogen Identification Policy: A Statement of Science as a Basis of Policy, Section 2: Methods for Estimating Cancer Risks from Exposure to Carcinogens. (Sacramento: Health and Welfare Agency)

38. Crump, KS, Guess, HA and Deal, KL (1977). Confidence intervals and test of hypotheses concerning dose response relations inferred from animal carcinogenicity data. Biometrics, 33, 437-51

39. Carlborg, FW (1979). Cancer, mathematical models and aflatoxin. Food Cosmet Toxicol, 17, 159-66

40. Anon (1981). Re-examination of the ED 01 Study Review of Statistics: The need for realistic statistical models for risk assessment. Fund Appl Toxicol, 1, 123-6

41. Purchase, IFH (1985). Formaldehyde: how serious is the risk to pathologists. Bull Roy Coll Pathol, 50, 4-8

42. Squire, RA (1981). Ranking animal carcinogens: a proposed regulatory approach. Science, 214,877-80

43. Pitot, HC (1980). Relationship of bioassay data on chemicals to their toxic and carcinogenic risk for humans. In Demopoulos, HB and Mehlman, MA (eds), Cancer and the Environment. pp. 431-50. (Washington: Pathotox)

44. Munro, IC and Krewski,DR (1981). Risk assessment and regulatory decision making. Food Cosmet, Toxicol, 19, 549-60

45. Ramsey, JC,Park, CN,Ott, MG and Gehring, PJ (1979). Carcinogenic risk assessment: ethylene dibromide. Toxicol Appl Pharmacol, 47, 411-14

46. Clayson, WB,Krewski,D and Munro, I (1985). Toxicological Risk Assessment, Vol. II: General Criteria and Case Studies. (Florida: CRC Press)

47. ECETOC (1982). Hepatocarcinogenesis in Laboratory Rodents: Relevance for Man. (Brussels: European Chemical Industry Ecology and Toxicology Centre, Monograph No. 4)

48. ECETOC (1982). RiskAssessmentof OccupationalChemical Carcinogens. (Brussels: European Chemical Industry Ecology and Toxicity Centre, Monograph No. 3)

49. Haseman, JK (1985). Issues in carcinogenicity testing: dose selection. Fund Appl Toxicol, 5, 66-78

50. Morton, DB andGriffiths, PHM (1985). Guidelines on the recognition of pain,distress and discomfort in experimental animals and an hypothesis for assessment. Vet Rec, 116, 431-6

51. Ames,BN(1983). Dietary carcinogens and anticarcinogens - oxygen radicals and degenerative diseases. Science, 221, 1256-63

52. Grasso, P (1983). Carcinogens in food. In Conning, DM and Lansdown, ABG (eds) Toxic Hazards inFood. pp. 122-44. (London: Croom Helm)

53. Shank, RC (ed.) (1981). Mycotoxins and N-Nitroso Compounds: Environmental Risks, Vol. I. (Florida: CRC Press)

54. Forbes, P (1985). The natural way to chemical warfare. New Sci, 1461, 27

55. Einhellig, FA (1985). Allelopathy - a natural protection, allochemicals. In Mandave, N (ed.) Handbook ofNatural Pesticides: Methods. Vol. I, pp. 161-200. (Florida: CRC Press)

56. Stich, HF (ed)(1983). Carcinogensand Mutagensinthe Environment, Vol. III: Naturally OccurringCompounds: Epidemiology and Distribution. (Florida: CRC Press)

57. National Research Council (1982). Diet, Nutrition and Cancer. (Washington: National Academy Press)

10
Cosmetics, Toiletries and Household Products

N. VAN ABBÉ

The diverse range of raw materials used in manufacturing cosmetics, toiletries and household products is encountered by vast numbers of people over the years, irrespective of age, sex or state of health. Exposure is often prolonged and repeated frequently, in some instances throughout a major part of the lifespan, mostly without medical or other expert supervision. Such a pattern of exposure in all the more advanced countries of the world seldom, in practice, gives rise to overt safety problems of any consequence or to insidious and possibly more serious adverse effects, according to the available evidence. Predictive safety evaluation based on experimental investigation is relatively new to the scene; the earlier way of selecting ingredients by a process of trial-and-error evidently functioned remarkably well on the whole. Inevitably mistakes were made now and again. For example, distinctly hazardous substances such as arsenic, mercury and atropine found their way into cosmetics at certain times but ingredients mostly seem to have been chosen at least partly for their inherent blandness, thereby providing quite an effective safeguard.

For a long time, potentially dangerous substances such as phenol, caustic soda and hypochlorite have featured regularly in the group of domestic cleansing and hygiene preparations classed as "household products". Surprisingly, though, accidental poisoning has never really been a widespread problem associated with the presence of such preparations in the home. The good sense of manufacturers, retailers and the lay public apparently ensures that a wide variety of products is kept and handled at home with sufficient care to account for their generally satisfactory record of safety-in-use. Some credit must also be accorded to various regulatory and control measures, although most of these have only come into existence quite recently.

Risks associated with using consumer products could unfortunately increase in the foreseeable future despite the growth of safety legislation, partly because some aspects of regulatory activity tend to encourage the development of more adventurous formulations. One reason for anticipating increased risk is that insistent demands for scientific evidence to support product advertizing claims may incidentally bring about a vigorous search for more efficacious products. Manufacturers may be expected to seek out ingredients with enhanced pharmacodynamic activity, which is likely to increase the chances of substantial toxic potential. The normal pressures of competition in mass markets might well be thought liable to generate a rather frantic demand for novel, if possibly toxic, ingredients. Legislative activity characteristic of the consumer era may, by insisting on product claims substantiation, underline the call for "active" ingredients which might be better avoided.

Even though nearly everyone would probably agree that cosmetics, toiletries and household products have an enviable record of safety-in-use, citing this favourable background in support of particular products or ingredients is clearly inadmissible. Attention would be focused, for example, on the possibility of a long interval between exposure and toxic responses and the fact that some delayed effects (e.g. chemical carcinogenesis) are usually hard to recognize. Failure to detect causal associations is certainly a danger in studying the epidemiological consequences of exposure to environmental chemicals of all kinds. As Doll[1] pointed out, however, the incidence of cancers unrelated to cigarette smoking has not escalated in recent years despite the twentieth-century "chemical explosion". Indeed, experience seems to show that carcinogenesis attributable to the chemical environment is relatively uncommon in the human species despite earlier fears to the contrary. Hence if there are no other grounds for suspicion, a long and apparently uneventful history of using an ingredient could justifiably be taken as a reasonable indication of lack of risk, even without firm data on the absence of delayed responses. The grounds for reaching a conclusion of this nature will never be incontrovertible, of course, but data from superficially more definitive laboratory studies are always subject to uncertainties of extrapolation.

Confidence may be increased if, for example, human experience is backed by favourable results from short-term genotoxicity studies. The main limitation is that epidemiological evidence is nearly always retrospective. This does not present a problem for reviewing the safety-in-use of an existing substance but a long record of safe use is inevitably missing when safety evaluation is needed on a new one. Meticulous attention should be given to any opportunity for observing human responses to, or tolerance towards, a new chemical, in view of the maximal relevance of such observations. Evidence reflecting the experience of process workers engaged in chemical synthesis may, for example, be far more informative than many exacting, costly and time-consuming laboratory investigations.

Apropos future requirements for predictive safety evaluation, an important factor is that the skin, under real-life conditions, provides quite a good protective barrier against a variety of chemical insults. Permeability of the skin may be readily demonstrated in the laboratory but the barrier property in practice must be credited with ensuring that topical exposure is usually well tolerated and nothing like as hazardous, for example, as exposure by the oral route. A major factor is that care in selecting ingredients and in their blending - in other words, the formulator's professional skill - has been and will surely continue to be a crucial safeguard. Predictive safety evaluation would be far more costly and speculative in the absence of a responsible approach to ingredient selection.

Long experience in the cosmetics and allied fields of the safety-in-use of typical ingredients and formulations is largely reassuring, but the regulatory trend sometimes appears to reflect a totally different scene. In many countries, and within supranational institutions like the EEC, a spate of new regulations has emerged mostly designed, so it seems, to protect the public against what must surely be described as no more than hypothetical hazards. Foreseeable consequences of "over-regulation" may include a heavy burden of financial cost which is sure to fall on consumers, a brake on product innovation and a substantial waste of scientific manpower and facilities, along with extensive and unnecessary use of laboratory animals.

Legislative zeal may perhaps be influenced partly by the supposedly low level of technical or scientific skill needed for carrying on business in the cosmetics and related fields. This may be voiced along the lines that there is no great enthusiasm for more stringent measures to exercise control over the major industrial concerns with their relatively generous research and quality assurance provisions. It is argued, though, that many smaller firms do not have adequate technical facilities. On such theoretical grounds, and on the pretext of a few isolated though not really very serious incidents, an array of controls, committees and testing requirements has come into being at a substantial cost in money and manpower. Whether this will ever succeed in preventing severe injury or loss of life is questionable, and unfortunately cannot be established with certainty. In theory the less expert manufacturers might have been tempted to take unjustifiable risks in the absence of legal constraints, but in reality they are more likely to emulate what is done by the major companies backed by their greater resources. Ingredient suppliers often exert a restraining influence on product manufacturers too, for the sake of their own reputations, and this will sometimes include steps to discourage the imprudent proliferation of new uses for chemical specialities.

Wherever there is anything akin to the Common Law in Britain, a governing principle will usually be that each individual manufacturer is held directly liable for damage caused by his products. Such a corollary to Article 2 of the EEC Cosmetics Directive, 1976[2] is not always easily enforced, however, because enforcement has to be preceded by the lodging of a claim. Experience shows that perseverance in serving notice of claims and going through with subsequent litigation varies greatly at different times and in different countries.

When product safety assurance is based on the user's right to claim damages if things go wrong, each manufacturer is prompted to erect a system of defences against possible charges of negligence, by acquiring extensive safety data with an accompanying likelihood of widespread duplication among different users of the same ingredients. Self-interest, however, does encourage some major manufacturers to counteract the massive cost of avoidable duplication by sharing information and even by collaborative research in trade associations, research associations and similar bodies. Vociferous objections to animal experimentation, whatever their intrinsic merits, run the risk of discouraging publication of the results of such experimentation. An obvious consequence will be the repetition of essentially the same studies by others, in ignorance of the original work and its outcome. Unfortunately the overall effect is thus to **increase** the numbers of animals used. By way of contrast, however, an impressive effort involving the sharing of safety data has been under way in the USA. The Cosmetic Ingredient Review (CIR) was intiated by the Cosmetic, Toiletry and Fragrance Association and the CIR reports are undoubtedly of great value for many other fields of application, as well as for cosmetics. A comparable programme of a collaborative nature has been carried through by the Research Institute for Fragrance Materials (RIFM).

Voluntary self-regulation by cosmetic manufacturers, to which CIR makes an admirable contribution, tends to be advocated as an alternative to more explicit regulatory constraint along the lines of statutory lists of permitted ingredients (so-called "positive" lists). A "positive" listing approach came to be accepted several decades ago in the food industry, and beynational and international authorities, mainly perhaps because it offered a suitable way of regulating the use of various additives but did not interfere with the composition of foodstuffs in respect of their major constituents. Manufacturers seem to find it convenient to have authoritative backing for a number of ancillary ingredients such as antioxidants and emulsifiers. The trend towards "positive" lists embracing some of the most important ingredients in cosmetics and related products is quite another matter, not nearly so acceptable to industry. "Positive" listing tends to create serious problems for the regulatory agencies too, with respect to the logistic and other problems involved in scrutinizing masses of safety evaluation data. Hence the regulatory control of ingredients for cosmetics and related products may well require alternatives to the "positive list" approach in the reasonably near future.

Control has been imposed in some countries by giving the poisons information centres a major role in the registration of consumer products. These establishments, however, are likely to have staff with expertise primarily concerned with clinical toxicology and especially the problems associated with acute toxicity and drug interactions. Predictive safety evaluation, especially in relation to delayed or chronic changes such as cell-mediated allergy and chemical carcinogenesis, calls for a considerably different training and experience. Involvement of the poisons information centres in the present context must therefore be seen as largely anachronistic.

138

THE FUTURE

It is remarkable that anything remotely under suspicion of being "racist" or "sexist" has come in for severe criticism or even legal action within an exceptionally short space of time following generations of indifference. Attitudes are capable of being transformed with surprising alacrity and a much wider variety of entrenched or cherished ideas and habits may also be overturned in the next decade or two. Styles of facial make-up and hair management normally tend to evolve rather slowly and steadily, but radically new developments could be superimposed on this gradual pattern of change at any time. For example, attitudes throughout the past hundred years towards the relative importance of women's and men's cosmetics might be greatly modified or even overturned!

Cosmetics and toiletries to accompany and to complement the vagaries of fashions in clothing a few years hence naturally defy prediction. Household products are correspondingly responsive to various influencing factors, such as the relative cost of DIY renovation compared to using paid craftsmen or to moving house, and they too are sensitive to technological advances . . . the availability, for example, of new resin polymers for formulating adhesives or of active constituents for household bleaches or garden insecticides. Until ballpoint pens were invented there was no market for products to remove the stains they sometimes leave behind; interdependence of this nature between consumer products makes it impossible to discuss future safety evaluation requirements in great detail. Some consumer products arise by way of trail-blazing innovation through original research or design improvement, but many depend on invention or technological advances originating in altogether different fields. Since further acceleration in technology is to be expected in future years, parallel developments in most kinds of consumer products are sure to follow. Without some insight into the characteristics of forthcoming new products or how they might be used, however, neither the nature of potential hazards nor the requirements for predictive safety evaluation are foreseeable.

Unlike ingredients and prescription medicines, the systems of regulatory control in most countries have so far avoided explicitly requiring cosmetics and related consumer products to be tested in the laboratory to show whether they may be used safely. The dossier system in France, however, could be regarded as an initial, tentative step along this road and consumerist spokesmen may from time to time argue persuasively or, at least, passionately in favour of compulsory testing. The heart of the matter is that life and risks are inseparable; civilized living has to reconcile many conflicting factors, and risk acceptability is a matter for individual and collective judgement. Nevertheless some kind of serious incident or emergency involving a new cosmetic, toiletry or household product could readily bring forth a demand for testing out of all proportion to the true level of risk in ordinary circumstances.

Whereas genuine alarm engendered by actual and serious harm to users is understandable, less rational anxiety is generated now and again by observations recorded in a laboratory study, not in actual use of a product. Conditions of experiment never reproduce precisely the conditions of exposure in normal use and the exposed populations (human, animal or even isolated cells) necessarily differ from the typical spectrum of purchasers. In other words, experimental observations rarely if ever justify a panic response. The cosmetics and toiletries field is peculiarly at risk of emotive and alarmist treatment by the lay media, especially as the products may always be denigrated as "trivial" compared to those that are more obviously essential. The lay media sometimes receive encouragement in a highly reprehensible way from scientists willing to abandon the established practice of first presenting their findings to be refereed before publication in the scientific press. No doubt a genuine need exists for society to have early warning of major unforeseen health hazards, but an equally important requirement is to avoid false alarms liable to blunt the keen edge of public responsiveness to real danger. The procedure of peer review and scientific publication, meant to give others an opportunity to verify the original observations, has stood the test of time and cannot be said to have drastically impeded scientific advance. This procedure possibly seems rather sluggish in the light of today's fast-moving needs but a likely outcome of overthrowing the system could well be to destroy the credibility of the media and also of the scientists concerned.

As an extension perhaps of the French dossier system, new arrangements may be envisaged whereby consumer products such as cosmetics would, by law, have to undergo a specified and extensive range of safety tests before release for sale. Alternatively release might depend on the award of a licence following detailed official scrutiny of formulae, safety testing data and possibly other kinds of information. Onerous requirements on these lines could surely be contemplated seriously for most kinds of consumer products only as the aftermath of some sort of catastrophe which is hard to imagine. The financial burden, the sacrifice of many more animals and the hindrance to normal, legitimate commercial activity would otherwise by wholly indefensible. Potent medicaments are, by nature, much more prone to be seriously toxic than cosmetic and similar products; testing requirements and formula scrutiny necessary for the former are never likely to be appropriate for the latter.

The description "household products" does not refer to a category of goods subject to precise definition and may, for example, embrace anything from an air freshener to a rat poison. Common sense is obviously needed in order to decide what potential risks need taking into account, or when these might reach an unacceptable level. Fortunately experience seems to suggest that household products are, on the whole, stored and used quite sensibly in practice. It is interesting to recall the approach taken by the Poisons Board[3] which came into being in Britain consequent upon passage of the Pharmacy and Poisons Act, 1933. The Board from time to time decided whether the sale of particular substances, some of which were or might have been present in household and other kinds of product, needed to be restricted or prohibited. A "negative list" scheme was adopted along with the pronouncement of restrictions or special cautionary labelling requirements in some instances where outright prohibition was not considered necessary. The UK Poisons List, reflecting the Board's deliberations, served a useful purpose for several decades; the wisdom of its provisions was indeed acknowledged when Annex II of the EEC Cosmetics Directive, 1976[2] was so obviously modelled on this List.

From the standpoint of predictive safety evaluation, a distinction may be drawn between testing ingredients or formulated products. On theoretical grounds there are undoubtedly reasons, at least in some circumstances, for recognizing that the blending together of ingredients in a formulation may alter the toxic effects due to the individual constituents (favourably or unfavourably). Generally, blending would be expected to modify rates of absorption, for example, rather than influencing the manifestation of fundamental toxic properties, e.g. carcinogenic potency, of a substance. Hence it will usually be considered important to understand the toxic potential of raw materials in detail but necessary only, perhaps, to undertake much more limited verification of potential safety-in-use in the case of a formulation. Certainly the present-day tendency is to permit or prohibit use of individual substances as raw materials (subject to reservations as to product purpose in some instances) without reference to any individual formulation. Nevertheless the EEC Cosmetics Directive imposes an overriding requirement in Article 2 to the effect that a **product** must not cause harm to health, irrespective of any testing or approval of **ingredients** specified in the Directive or elsewhere. A provision of this type is being incorporated into the legislation of member states, and in any case this has much the same implications as existing liabilities under Common Law. In effect, a manufacturer may be at fault even when using nothing but approved ingredients, unless proper steps have been taken to consider exposure levels, for example, or to examine possible interactions, chemical or physiological, between the ingredients in a particular formulation. In other words, inclusion of a substance in a "positive list" should not be taken as carte blanche to incorporate it into a product. This might be interpreted as implying that predictive safety evaluation is needed for all formulated products, but such a view has not been proclaimed and upheld in any Court of Law at the time of writing.

Difficulties must be expected at times through ignorance of the likely end-uses for a prospective raw material at the time it is undergoing safety evaluation. As some of the foreseeable uses would probably involve significant exposure systemically, however, a chemical manufacturer often puts a new substance through a broad safety screening; this is also liable to be necessary for Health and Safety at Work reasons in order to safeguard process workers who may come in contact with the new chemical. Cosmetic and other end-uses not too much concerned with systemic exposure are naturally able to take advantage of the information generated. Even though the data may not be directly relevant for topical exposure, access to the results of a broad screening programme is reassuring if the findings are essentially favourable. Information derived from systemic exposure, however, will not necessarily be acceptable in lieu of data for percutaneous absorption and toxicity, in the case of ingredients liable to be repeatedly applied liberally over a substantial area and left in situ, sometimes day after day. Percutaneous toxicity is so closely associated with toxicokinetic considerations (first-pass metabolism and rate of excretion versus rate of absorption) that it may show no real similarity to peroral toxicity. If, however, percutaneous **toxicity** has been shown by means of simple test procedures to be minimal, the case for a separate study of percutaneous **absorption** (which would be far more costly and time-consuming) must surely have been dispelled.

Although there may be good reason to require details concerning percutaneous absorption and toxicity for an ingredient or product to be applied over a relatively wide area of the skin and left there for many hours, a much more relaxed approach is usually appropriate for a material largely rinsed away during normal use, such as a toilet soap or shampoo. There may be grounds for more concern where an ingredient is known to be adsorbed strongly on to the skin, but binding to or adsorption on hair would possibly reduce rather than augment systemic exposure. Household products of some kinds, such as disinfectants, do not normally come in contact with the tissues at all and their safety evaluation would rationally need to be concerned only with the possible risk of occasional accidental exposure by various routes.

PROSPECTS FOR SAFETY EVALUATION

Limitation of exposure nearly always diminishes toxic risk. For studying the potential toxicity of a medicine, other than a topical application, systemic exposure is appropriately considered in terms of the total dose administered, and risk estimates may be derived from the observed dose/response behaviour. Similarly, safety margins for food additives are calculated on the basis of systemic exposure to the expected total dietary intake. However, in the case of topically applied substances (whether these are medicaments or cosmetics), systemic exposure is not usually intended. With household products such exposure is invariably unintentional. Unfortunately, however, factual information about the actual levels of systemic exposure, if any, to non-medicinal and non-food environmental chemicals is rarely available. In consequence, regulatory agencies tend to "err on the safe side" and to examine the toxicity data in relation to distinctly "pessimistic" exposure calculations. Hence there may be more to gain in future by generating reliable information on systemic exposure to consumer products than by any other steps concerned with improving the means of predicting safety-in-use. This would seem to be valid from the standpoint both of consumers and manufacturers. Striving towards the more sensitive detection of toxicity seems a little ridiculous when true levels of systemic exposure may be several orders of magnitude different from present-day suppositions.

With cosmetics, toiletries and household products, the most likely safety problems in their normal use are concerned with skin irritancy, type IV or delayed cell-mediated contact sensitization, eye irritancy and, mainly for spray products, inhalation toxicity. Other forms of toxicity occasionally give rise to problems and call for a wider range of studies with particular ingredients or products. For example, contact urticaria sometimes causes difficulty and introduces a need for special predictive testing. In the European context it has yet to be seen to what extent the notification requirements of the Sixth Amendment to the EEC Dangerous Substances Directive[4] will in practice ensure that an adequate range of toxicological studies is on file for a potential new ingredient. Where chemical suppliers foresee a sufficient demand for new substances to justify investment in the testing required under the Sixth Amendment, this is likely to be advantageous for cosmetic manufacturers and other users. Sometimes, perhaps often, suppliers may be convinced that new raw materials will simply not be worth pursuing commercially, especially if potential clients are likely to require only relatively small quantities. The impact of contemporary legislation on the availability of speciality chemicals may take several years to reach some kind of equilibrium.

At the time of writing, the latest Home Office report to Parliament in the UK[5] shows that safety testing of cosmetics and allied products accounts for only some 0.5% of all living animal experimentation within the meaning of the existing law. The numbers of animals so used is, of course, a much smaller proportion compared with the numbers of animals used as food. The statistics undoubtedly mean that in Britain the vast majority of new or modified cosmetics, toiletries and household products entering the consumer market are not tested on living animals at all. Escalating costs of raw materials, which manufacturers try to avoid passing on to consumers, and strong competitive pressures certainly foster a programme of reformulating and relaunching even the most well-established brands at relatively short intervals. Whatever testing is thought to be needed and is actually done, however, the Home Office returns clearly imply that new versions of these products hardly ever undergo live animal testing. Presumably, in most instances, the ingredients have all been safely used before and the manufacturers, after consulting the background data, consider either that further testing is unnecessary or that human volunteer studies are feasible and will be most informative. Exceptions where animal testing is carried out are the small number of formulations containing radically new ingredients, those which are specially meant for use on babies or small children and in a few instances those destined for overseas markets where animal testing is a legislative requirement.

At the present time substantial efforts are being made in many quarters to identify so-called "alternatives" to the use of living animals. Biological scientists tend to regard live animal studies as an important, though not always infallible, source of essential information; nevertheless, many would undoubtedly prefer on humane grounds to avoid using living animals. The tendency to move away from living animals to speedier, cheaper and more reliable in vitro techniques is well illustrated, for example, in the universal change to such methods for vitamin assay in place of the earlier in vivo techniques. The successful elaboration of "alternative" methods obviating the need for living animals has not been at all easy in many areas of potential interest. Reproducibility between different laboratories, relevance and sensitivity of the methods are important requirements. When the scientific foundations have been well laid and there are clear financial benefits to be gained, enthusiasm to take up "alternatives" is by no means lacking; this is particularly evident in the wide acceptance and use of in vitro bacterial mutagenicity testing. Worldwide attention to the development of "alternative" methods must surely bear fruit in other directions too before long.

The elimination of live animal testing is a desirable objective but there will still be a great need for safety predictions that are thoroughly dependable with respect to human use of various products. The most useful answers may well come, however, by way of new techniques using human volunteers rather than laboratory animals or in vitro systems of one kind or another. To be realistic, the permissible range of toxicity testing on volunteers is not limitless. There are bound to be restrictions, for example, on the extent of acute toxicity evaluation or the severity of eye lesions that could be inflicted. On the other hand, confidence must surely be maximized whenever a safety prediction is the outcome of a study using human volunteers. An important consideration is that exposure levels in volunteer studies may legitimately be reduced by at least an order of magnitude compared to studies on other species without detracting from the reliability of the findings. One way to minimize any risk involved in using volunteers is to improve the sensitivity with which adverse changes may be detected; great progress has already been made in introducing comparable improvements in the analysis of blood and tissue levels, and it is to be hoped that physiological monitoring will also become much more sensitive and informative. Reconsideration of some long-standing ethical concepts may also be needed, e.g. concerning the use of human volunteers in eye irritancy studies, but only with great care to avoid sacrificing the progress made since 1945 in safeguarding the interests of patients and volunteers.

Just as there are bound to be limits to the versatility of volunteer studies, too much should not be expected of in vitro techniques. Studies on isolated cells or tissues, for example, can never be expected to reproduce all the complex interactions shown by a whole multicellular organism. Many physiological processes may be subdivided into component parts amenable to study in vitro, however, and this type of approach is often worthwhile despite the obvious limitations. To be really successful, a novel in vitro test procedure needs to offer a relatively rapid and inexpensive means of showing whether definitive in vivo studies (e.g. with human volunteers) will be likely to yield satisfactory findings. In other words the most effective "alternative" methods so far, in the toxicological field, have been those which are useful as screening procedures and it may well be better to aim initially in this direction rather than seeking to replace in vivo procedures entirely. Thus, it is virtually impossible to envisage an in vitro test capable of giving 100% reassurance of the absence of teratogenic potential. Nevertheless, a great deal of time and money, as well as many animals, could be spared if it were possible to demonstrate convincingly in vitro that only perhaps three out of a group of twenty new chemicals would be worth submitting to in vivo testing with reasonable prospects of favourable results. Bearing in mind that numerous proposals for the adoption of novel in vitro tests may reasonably be expected to come from the extensive laboratory work in progress, it will be important to see that these are indeed brought into effective use without delay, and this would seem most likely if they prove sufficiently reliable to serve as preliminary screening tests prior to human volunteer studies.

SOME PARTICULAR NEEDS

In terms of a pressing requirement for new methodology in the safety evaluation of topically applied substances, first thoughts centre on the prediction of Type IV allergic sensitizing potential. For a new compound, the present-day approach is almost entirely limited to one of the various guinea-pig sensitization tests and/or some form of human repeated insult patch test. Both are capable of identifying the more powerful sensitizers, but neither is fully satisfactory in its reliability for detecting weak allergens. Apart from particular problems of methodology, undesirable features are the need to use animals with consequent problems of interspecies extrapolation or to incur the risk of long-term sensitizing of human volunteers through failure to conduct sufficient preliminary testing. Extensive fundamental studies of the immune mechanism are in hand, however, and better understanding is already becoming available[6]. The detection of sensitizing potential wholly by in vitro methods may not be an immediate prospect but ways and means could well evolve before long as a logical outcome of the on-going research.

It is often decided that there is no need to study sensitizing potential on a product formulation because satisfactory data are already available for all the ingredients. The underlying assumptions will, however, be invalidated if there is any likelihood of enhancement of sensitizing properties in a particular blend of ingredients. Little is known of this type of risk and a real need exists for more information. It is commonly assumed that quantitive aspects of the risk of eliciting a sensitization response are not important but, in fact, the use of potential sensitizers at concentrations below those needed for eliciting a response may well be quite satisfactory in many circumstances.

The in vitro prediction of skin sensitizing potential offers a relatively self-contained target, perhaps only a jump or two ahead of existing knowledge. In vitro predictive methods for studying ocular toxicity, percutaneous absorption and photo-activated skin reactions are probably farther away and some aspects of toxicology, such as testing for teratogenic potential, show no clear signs so far of being amenable to an in vitro approach at all. Even though in vitro predictive approaches fundamentally sound in scientific terms may not be near at hand, the requirements might still be partly fulfilled in the meantime by empirical methods. For example, in vitro techniques giving reasonably satisfactory correlation with in vivo eye irritancy might well serve a useful purpose as a preliminary screen and their development certainly deserves to be encouraged.

An important principle to which Scaife[7] drew attention is

that a new test should not be judged primarily according to how well the results correlate with a previous laboratory method; since the purpose is nearly always to predict safety-in-use for human subjects, correlation should in principle be related to toxic changes in humans. There is little merit in assessing an innovative approach by making comparisons which, in effect, only perpetuate the problems of interpretation associated with its forerunner. To be specific, a new skin sensitization test really needs to be compared with, or calibrated against, human skin sensitization and a proposed eye irritancy test against human eye irritancy. Difficulties abound but they should not be insurmountable.

Data on percutaneous absorption may be required for any biologically active compound liable to be applied repeatedly to relatively large skin areas and left in situ without rinsing. If the compound under consideration is known to display only negligible toxicity by various routes of administration, however, there would seem to be little reason to study its percutaneous absorption. Typical absorption studies using rodents, for example, have utilized radioisotope (usually C-14) labelling of the compound being examined, followed by autoradiography of the skin or even the whole body along with blood, tissue, urine and faeces counts of radioactivity. Carefully controlled radiotracer studies using human volunteers may also be feasible, subject to careful scrutiny of the ethical considerations involved, even though the absorption studies are intended for "non-essential" purposes such as the study of cosmetic ingredients. Human volunteer studies on percutaneous absorption tend to be rather costly but they are likely to be much more convincing than any others, including in vitro experiments with excised human skin or in vivo animal studies.

Modern instrumental methods for "cold" analysis, such as HPLC and GC-MS, help to provide a degree of sensitivity approaching in some measure that of radiotracer techniques. There may also be advantages in studying absorption by making use of stable, non-radioactive, isotopes. The administration of compounds enriched (up to perhaps 90%) with stable isotopes such as C-13, N-15 or O-18 poses virtually no risk to volunteers beyond any risk due to the unlabelled compound, and may facilitate monitoring of distribution and excretion as well as absorption. Unfortunately it does not follow that H-2 enrichment (deuteration) will always provide such reliable data or be as hazard-free, since there could be a greater risk of changes in enzyme kinetics. Radiotracer techniques are still likely to be the most sensitive, and will be the first choice if there are not likely to be any major ethical problems; choice will also be influenced by the availability of labelled intermediate compounds from which the radiotracer labelled or stable isotope-enriched test compound may be synthesized.

Percutaneous absorption is an area of toxicological interest which might reasonably be thought suitable for mathematical modelling or computer simulation. Although a moderate degree of optimism may be warranted in terms of the prediction of absorption per se, a comprehensive pharmacokinetic approach has to consider distribution, metabolism and excretion too, and provide an insight into the possible risk of accumulation in the body. The extensive background knowledge essential for quantitative prediction of these kinetic factors or to forecast tissue storage emphasizes the need for caution in developing a purely mathematical approach.

Photoactivated biological responses are sometimes especially troublesome, and predictive methods none too satisfactory. Many compounds which absorb in the UV spectral region are potentially capable of initiating photo-reactions in the skin. Although special tests for phototoxic and photo-sensitizing potential are available, their pesticide reliability does not warrant a high degree of confidence; this is particularly worrying because chronic actinic hypersensitivity can be a serious disability. A tribute should, however, be paid to collaborative efforts under the aegis of the Research Institute for Fragrance Materials (RIFM) and the International Fragrance Association (IFRA). An example has been concerned with the photosensitizing properties of nitro-musks in shaving lotions[8]. Useful empirical answers have emerged, even though much more probably remains to be learned.

The level of distress or discomfort associated with using a cosmetic or toiletry product is not necessarily in proportion to the real health risk involved. A painful stinging sensation is a relatively frequent problem, for example, with aftershaves and some antiperspirants. Living epidermis and an intact nerve supply are presumably unavoidable for investigating the stinging problem, and human volunteer studies would seem most likely to allow the necessary monitoring of subjective responses. In most circumstances, painful responses to applied substances probably involve the release from neighbouring tissues of chemical mediators capable of stimulating sensory receptors. Identification of the mediators might provide the basis for an in vitro and perhaps even a quantitative method of predictive testing; the significance of prostaglandin production in various tissues in response to ethanol has been described[9]. Another difficulty occasionally encountered is the occurrence of a miliaria-like condition of the skin sometimes designated as "pomade acne", allegedly attributable to the occlusive or irritant effect of various oily or greasy applications. As the microanatomy peculiar to human skin is likely to be closely involved, this appears to be another case for human volunteer studies.

Earlier it was mentioned that inhalation toxicity deserves attention. The typical problems associated with acute or chronic systemic toxicity related to inhalational exposure are, with some exceptions, relatively well-established. However, a field of interest specially relevant in connection with various consumer products is the prediction of adverse reactions to the inhalation of finely divided particles, which assumes greater importance when a substantial number are in a size range appropriate for alveolar exposure. Alleged health hazards in recent years were concerned with the possible inhalation of hair spray resins and also cosmetic talc. The substantial efforts that were devoted to resolving these questions should help to minimize any future health problems arising with other products that may give rise to fine particulate matter when they are used in the home. Short-term screening methods to identify potentially hazardous new materials will be needed. An approach embodying both particle size analysis and in vitro cytotoxicity testing[10] looks promising. Inhalation hazards such as occupational asthma, possibly in association with hypersensitivity to cosmetics and related products in a work environment, may also require further attention.

Questions are sometimes raised with regard to inhalation toxicity aspects of the propellants used in pressurized aerosol products for cosmetic and household purposes and, in particular, about the halogenated hydrocarbons used in this way. It would certainly be unwise to use any compound as an aerosol propellant without good background data on its short- and long-term toxicity. In addition, consideration may need to be given to possible idiosyncratic responses, e.g. exceptional sensitivity to haloalkanes in mature individuals with some degree of cardiac impairment.

Safety evaluation problems also arise in connection with organic solvents in the liquid state coming into contact with the tissues, as well as by vapour inhalation. With cosmetics, for example, this applies to solvents for nail enamel and with household products examples abound, such as in paint strippers, adhesives, sealants and grease-spot removers. Since the requirement for such uses is unlikely to be considered sufficient in economic terms to justify the wide and costly range of toxicological investigations needed to validate a new solvent with respect to possible systemic hazards, it seems almost certain that only those solvents which have been thoroughly studied for other purposes will be considered for cosmetic and related uses. Even so, the available data will need careful scrutiny, and detailed attention will probably have to be given to potential topical hazards. Often the defatting action of an organic solvent could be injurious to the skin to a greater or lesser degree, and the possibility of skin allergy may not have been previously studied.

A further problem has emerged in recent years owing to the widespread use of volatile organic solvents, especially by way of deliberate inhalation under conditions of restricted ventilation, often by adolescents or children. At present it is virtually impossible to predict which solvents will prove to have serious abuse potential, and it is also difficult to be sure what degree of toxic risk will become manifest in practice (as distinct from the risk of asphyxia). Hence it is hard to advise on the choice of solvents for formulations of various kinds in such a way as to minimize toxic hazard if they are subsequently used for "sniffing". Awareness of the need for a predictive technique to detect solvent abuse potential should eventually lead to positive suggestions, but answers have so far proved elusive and interim control measures will doubtless be essential. Retailers of relevant goods may well be the first responsible individuals to encounter abuse of or addiction to new solvent-containing products (e.g. through seeing unexpectedly frequent repeat purchasing or irrational behaviour in the shop), and might be encouraged to set in motion an alerting system. This might be effective sooner than a notification scheme relying wholly on the medical profession, which tends mainly to see the late or serious cases once abuse or addiction is too well established for countermeasures to be easily employed.

CONCLUSIONS

The well-being of consumers and the commercial viability of a manufacturer are both likely to be affected by the way in which pass or fail decisions are reached on various substances or products in relation to their anticipated safety-in-use. Inappropriate decisions would be liable to have dangerous or expensive consequences. Criteria for the acceptability of safety data (especially those concerning topical effects) have often been based on arbitrary levels of toxicity, and always run the risk of introducing misconceptions, e.g. as a result of using non-linear scoring scales to record adverse changes. Bioassayists long ago came to appreciate the benefit of using internationally standardized reference materials to serve as simultaneous controls. The use of standard preparations in bio-assays tended to go out of fashion, however, when precise instrumental techniques became available for many assay purposes, but the principle remains. Indeed it would often be helpful to examine the biological activity of a prospective new product or new chemical by direct simultaneous comparison with its predecessor or some similar material with a well-established safety performance if, as frequently happens, an absolute level of human risk cannot be determined. For such purposes, predictive value may be optimized by avoiding experimental conditions leading either to zero or to severe responses, i.e. it is obviously best to use the most nearly linear region of an assessment scale, whether this is subjective or objective and strictly parametric or not. Such criteria apply especially to cosmetics and toiletries, as the dose-response pattern for possible inflammatory changes is not usually linear under severe conditions.

There is a temptation in some quarters, perhaps, to imagine that ever more pressing demands for safety testing could be introduced without giving any thought to consequent effects on the prices consumers will have to pay. This fallacy has been discussed in a UK Government White Paper[11] thus:

> In safety, as in other fields, there does, however, come a point where additional benefits begin to become disproportionately expensive. Safety policy must reflect a judgement on the degree to which the community as a whole is prepared to pay for additional safety. The Government has not pursued suggestions which would involve major interference with the normal processes of manufacture and trade and so put up unduly the prices which consumers have to pay for their products.

Despite the natural inclination to see the future of predictive safety evaluation primarily in relation to Western needs, there must surely be considerable scope for improving the safety-in-use of consumer products indigenous to the less developed so-called Third World countries. Different raw materials and different standards of purity may well apply. The import of cosmetics to supply ethnic minorities in Britain drew attention, for example, to abnormal risks of heavy-metal poisoning. Undoubtedly it will not be easy to find the resources for predictive safety testing in many densely populated territories burdened already with chronic financial problems. In such places most people obviously could not afford to purchase imported Western consumer products to benefit from their high standards. Help may be required on an international scale, and indeed is already provided by the World Health Organization in a limited way. Studying the nature and range of consumer safety problems in various territories calls for priority attention, as it will be virtually impossible to devise effective countermeasures without reliable background knowledge.

A compromise of some kind always has to be reached between testing for every conceivable risk that might accompany exposure to a product or raw material and the effort worth making for this purpose. Scientific, economic, legal and ethical factors are all involved to varying degrees over the course of time. The chances of elaborating a totally infallible system of predictive testing for any kind of product are slender. The wide range of problems, and the state of the art scientifically, all suggest a long-term need for good sense accompanied by readiness to shoulder personal responsibility for decisions taken in the light of such data as are available. Safety evaluation always has to culminate in a judgement reached by individuals. There is no prospect that matrix schemes, checklists or computerized data handling will ever take the place of thinking biological scientists paying heed to their own experience and intuitive reasoning. They need the help of up-to-date, well-validated methodology to reach satisfactory conclusions, and there is a great deal of scope for developing less costly, quicker, more humane and more reliable ways of reaching the necessary decisions. It will also be important to preserve a sense of proportion in relation to the inherent toxicity of various kinds of products; in the case of cosmetics and similar products their intrinsic biological inertness has been and, so far, still is, a powerful factor limiting the scale of predictive safety testing generally needed to safeguard the health of consumers.

REFERENCES

1. Doll, R (1977). Strategy for detection of cancer hazards to man. Nature, 265, 589
2. Official Journal of European Community (1976). L. 262/169 (76/768/EEC) Council Directive of 27 July 1976 on the Approximation of the Laws of the Member States Relating to Cosmetic Products
3. Dale, JR and Appelbe, GE (1983). Pharmacy Law and Ethics, 3rd edn, p. 175. (London: Pharmaceutical Press)
4. Official Journal of European Community (1979). L. 259/10 (79/831/EEC) Council Directive of 18 September 1979 Amending for the Sixth Time, Directive 67/548/EEC on the Approximation of the Laws, Regulations and Administrative Provisions Relating to the Classification, Packaging and Labelling of Dangerous Substances
5. HMSO (1984). Cmnd. 9311 Statistics of Experiments on Living Animals
6. Polak, L (1980). Current concept of allergic skin reactions.

Int J Cosmet Sci, 2, 251

7. Scaife, M (1982). An investigation of detergent action on cells in vitro and possible correlation with in vivo data. Int J Cosmet Sci, 4, 179

8. Cronin, E (1984). Photosensitivity to musk ambrette. Contact Dermatol, 11,88

9. Dubin, NH, Wolff, MC, Thomas, CL and Di Blasi, MC (1985). Prostaglandin production by rat vaginal tissue, in vitro, in response to ethanol, a mild mucosal irritant. Toxicol Appl Pharmacol, 78, 458

10. Davies, R, Skidmore, JW, Griffiths, DM and Moncrieff, CB (1983). Cytotoxicity of talc for macrophages in vitro. Fd Chem Toxicol, 21, 210

11. HMSO (1984). Cmnd. 9302, The Safety of Goods

11

Substances of Abuse

J. MARKS

Substance abuse is one of the major problems of our modern society, both in industrialized and developing nations. In the United States over the past 20 years there has been an epidemic of substance abuse (particularly narcotics, marijuana and cocaine). A similar epidemic is predicted for Europe and other industrially developed countries over the next few years as the American market is currently saturated and the drug pushers seek fresh fields.

There is, however, nothing new in man's dependence on pleasure-giving substances and activities. Man has long employed such substances in an attempt to banish pain and discomfort; to attain a state of oblivion, euphoria or ectasy; or to escape from unpleasant reality into a much more agreeable state of fantasy. The substances which are abused, and society's approach to them, varies with time and from one culture to another. The substances are themselves regarded as sacred by one culture but condemned as a devil's instrument by another, and their popularity has waxed and waned over the centuries.

Much of this field of study is still covered with confusion, not only because the socially acceptable practices of one generation or community are the legally enforceable abuses of another, but because much of the terminology is inconsistent. As Eddy et al.[1] have pointed out, almost any substance may be the subject of abuse,

> "There is scarcely any agent which can be taken into the body to which some individuals will not get a reaction satisfactory or pleasurable to them persuading them to continue its use even to the point of abuse."

TERMINOLOGY

Any of the understanding of the problems of drug abuse demands a clear definition of the terminology that is to be used, and the author has accepted the definition of the World Health Organization

(WHO, 1950[2]; 1969[3]). Among the WHO definitions there are some which are important for our present understanding.

1. **Drug dependence**: a state, psychic and sometimes also physical, resulting from the interaction between a living organism and a drug, characterized by behavioural and other responses that always include a compulsion to take the drug on a continuous or periodic basis in order to experience its psychic effects, and sometimes to avoid the discomfort of its absence. Tolerance may or may not be present. A person may be dependent on more than one drug.

2. **Abuse**: persistent or sporadic excessive drug use inconsistent with or unrelated to acceptable medical practice.

3. **Narcotic**: the general term narcotic covers those substances that relieve pain and induce sleep, whether they be naturally occurring substances, derivatives of such substances or synthetic substances. In the more specific sense they are defined as the drugs which are covered by the Single Convention on Narcotic Drugs 1961[4].

4. **Psychotropic**: any substance, natural or synthetic, which has the capacity to produce a state of dependence, exert central nervous system activity and lead to abuse which constitutes, or is likely to constitute, a public health and social problem and which is controlled under the Convention on Psychotropic Substances 1971[5].

FACTORS THAT LEAD TO PROBLEMS OVER APPROPRIATE TESTING METHODS

The difference between dependence during therapy and abuse

The classical picture of abuse in the socio-recreational scene is a combination of psychological and physical dependence coupled with tolerance such that the user rapidly escalates the dose. For many substances of dependence, tolerance and hence dose escalation is also a feature of dependence during therapeutic use. In these circumstances there is very little difference between dependence in therapy and socio-recreational abuse.

However for certain substances (e.g. the benzodiazepines) dependence in the therapeutic situation can occur with no obvious signs of tolerance and the dose is not escalated. On the other hand in the socio-recreational scene tolerance to these substances is still the rule and very high doses are taken[6].

Hence it would appear that the psychopathology of the two disorders differs significantly. It is therefore important to try to distinguish the two, or at least to decide whether one should be testing for dependence in the narrow sense or abuse risk in the wider sense.

Another related problem stems from the fact that a vast

154

number of therapeutic substances can lead to a rebound reaction on withdrawal[7]. The symptomatology varies with the pharmacological effect of the substance. Some of these substances have no known dependence potential. Equally the relationship between a rebound reaction and a withdrawal reaction with a drug of dependence is far from clear. It probably derives from the perceived symptomatology and the personality of the host. Hence the precise concept of dependence is sometimes unclear, which renders testing difficult.

The abuse "cascade" - variation between substances

It is widely held in lay circles that the abuse of one substance leads inevitably to the abuse of more powerful substances. In consequence it is maintained that it is important to avoid all possibility of such a cascade by banning all substances which may be subject to abuse.

It is true that for many substances of abuse it is possible to trace a movement from one substance to a more powerful one. This may not necessarily be the result of a pharmacological effect. It is important to stress that there is no evidence that substances such as caffeine, nicotine and alcohol, which are clearly substances of dependence and which can be abused[6], even if that abuse is socially acceptable, lead on to the use of any other drugs. Nor is there evidence that sedatives (e.g. barbiturates, benzodiazepine) or marijuana give rise to the use of harder drugs[8] (e.g. narcotics). Some drugs appear to encourage a drug "cascade", others not.

One of the inherent difficulties is that once a substance which can give rise to abuse is classed as illicit, it automatically encourages the movement of the user into the drug scene area. There is then a greater chance of cross-fertilization of ideas. Moreover use is encouraged by the fact that members of the group become pushers to find additional funds for their higher-priced drugs.

It is also important to appreciate that some substances are drugs of primary abuse, while others are usually only abused as a secondary consideration in the socio-recreational scene[6,9]. All these factors have particular relevance for the definition of the features which are relevant in dependence testing.

Multifactorial problem

The concept of a dependence-producing "capacity" or "potential" which resides in a drug itself has been questioned by some authorities in respect of drugs other than narcotics. They suggest that it is more relevant to speak of "dependence-prone individuals" who abuse a variety of substances and can develop dependence upon any or all of them. This has been described by Edwards[10] in the case of alcohol. It can equally be applied to other central nervous system depressants (barbiturates, non-barbiturate sedatives and tranquillizers).

It is apparent that within the field of psychostimulants and sedatives there is a contributory role exerted by the drug. Studies in animals and man have demonstrated clear evidence of physical and psychological dependence when large doses are given for a prolonged period[6,11-13]. Moreover clinical reports on at least some patients who have become dependent during therapy reveal a previously normal personality. Various attempts have been made to express the liability risk of substances in quantitative form[11]. Nevertheless it is clear that there are several factors that lead to dependence on a drug in which the nature of the drug is only one of the elements, the others including the individual himself and his environment[13]. The importance of environmental, personal and behavioural factors compared with pharmacological ones has been stressed by Fabre et al[14]. Berger[15] even goes so far as to say "there are no addictive drugs, only addictive people". Although this, in my opinion, overstates the situation, it does stress the multifactorial nature of the problem.

Dependence risk compared with abuse risk

From what has been said above, it follows that the risk of dependence does not necessarily equate with the level of abuse. The risk of dependence is itself a multifactorial problem and hence the risk varies from one person to another and from one time to another. Kielholz[16] has stressed the interplay which leads from drug ingestion to drug dependence.

Whether drug dependence leads on to drug abuse also depends upon several different factors, including the social environment, public attitudes and the personality of the individual. Hence, while it is broadly true that abuse of substances implies that they are drugs of dependence (exception for example marijuana), it is not necessarily true that drugs of dependence will always be subject to abuse in the community.

The development of abuse may depend upon such extraneous factors as technical knowledge. For example, "whereas addiction in chronic coca-leaf chewers among the natives of South America leads only infrequently to severe dependence (cocaism), the extracted cocaine is one of our strongest dependence-producing substances (cocainism) . . .[17].

Hence it is important to define whether one is trying to measure dependence risk or the risk of abuse and psychological dependence may be a more powerful stimulus to abuse potential than is physical dependence.

All these factors have particular relevance for the definition of the features which are relevant in dependence testing.

CURRENT SITUATION

Assessment of dependence liability

Two World Health Organization Expert Committees[12,13] have reviewed the techniques for evaluating the dependence potential of drugs in general. In addition the specific problem of the assessment of the dependence liability of psychotropic drugs was considered in the Twenty-first Report of the WHO Expert Committee on Drug Dependence[11]. Readers are advised to consult these publications for a detailed consideration of the techniques, their merits and problems. The present account only reviews the broad principles.

Both animal and human techniques are available though most of the animal studies relate more accurately to physical dependence. Since the methods used in animal research determine factors that may or may not be related to factors for human dependence, they must of course be correlated with human experience to ensure that they have clinical validity. Ultimately, of course, the risk of dependence in patients using drugs under therapeutic conditions can only be determined during normal clinical usage. However, experience has shown that some of the experimental methods appear to lead to valid assessment of the risk.

Animal studies

Despite the fact that the various substances demonstrate marked differences in their manifestations of dependence in man, animal tests for possible dependence follow a similar pattern for all substances.

A sine qua non of dependence production is that the substance shall exert an effect on the central nervous system. This can be demonstrated in single- and multiple-dose pharmacological studies. Such studies therefore form part of the testing procedure. Coupled with these pharmacological tests there can be biochemical investigations showing alteration of levels of transmitter substances (for example, the biogenic amines).

It is also valuable to examine the toxicological profile of the substance. Substances with unpleasant and immediate side-effects are less likely to be abused than those that do not show such properties.

During pharmacological studies various other phenomena commonly associated with dependence may become apparent. These include cross-tolerance with substances of known dependence liability; drug interactions; behaviour changes, particularly those of rapid onset; and rebound effects after stopping the drug.

Studies that suggest physical dependence liability can be divided into two classes: those in which the substance induces primary dependence in one or more animal species when administered on a chronic basis; and those in which the substance can be shown to substitute for one of known dependence liability in animals that have been made physically dependent on that agent. The present techniques were reviewed by Thompson and Unna[18]. The exact manifestations which indicate abstinence vary from one drug class to another. It is important to realize that physical dependence has so far only been **positively** established for drugs that show central nervous system depressant activity. Hence the tests described above have a limited role in the study of stimulants or hallucinogens.

Studies that suggest psychological dependence liability are based upon the view that substances that demonstrate psychological dependence in man show reinforcement of drug-seeking and drug-taking behaviour in animals. Hence the majority of animal studies to predict psychological dependence liability involve self-administration techniques. These have now been established for a variety of species including rats, cats, dogs and monkeys[11]. Most depend upon a lever-pressing stimulus for administration of the drug by intravenous or intragastric routes. Such reinforcing effects in animal studies have been demonstrated for both central nervous system depressants and stimulants, but the results are, to say the least, equivocal for hallucinogens.

As with the tests for physical dependence, so with the self-administration tests; the methods involve both primary progressive phenomena and cross-substitution. In some techniques the animals can choose between different drugs, so a preference rating for self-administration can be attempted. Of particular relevance to stimulant drugs are some of the drug discriminative procedures[19].

Although **hallucinogens** are classified with the dependence-producing drugs for legislation purposes, and are clearly drugs of abuse, there is little convincing evidence that they really have a dependence liability. It is therefore scarcely surprising that there are no clear predictive animal tests for these. Among the currently available drugs there is a measure of correlation between abnormal patterns of animal behaviour after drug administration and abuse potential in man, but there is no reason to believe that this would apply with new and further chemical classes of psychedelic drugs.

Human studies

Reports of adverse effects, including dependence, by their very nature, must be anecdotal in the first instance. Although experimental production of dependence in volunteers was undertaken in the past, there is a significant level of morbidity, and indeed mortality, with withdrawal of drugs of dependence. This precludes such studies on an experimental basis. Moreover, very high doses are usually required to provoke dependence within a reasonable time-span and the validity of the observations for practical therapeutics is therefore in doubt. The ethical considerations covering attempted substitution, reinforcement techniques and preference rating of research compounds in known addicts are less clear, but such methods would in any case only give information relative to known and recognized types of dependence, and not to a new class.

Current, natural medical and regulatory concern about dependence is likely to ensure that any compound with a dependence liability which manifests itself at the clinical trial stage either does not reach the market place or is subject to stringent controls. Hence in a practical therapeutic sense the dependence risk of new drugs is likely to be low, and mainly determined by medical practitioners in isolated patients after long-term therapeutic use. Different criteria apply in the socio-recreational situation.

FUTURE NEEDS AND PROBLEMS

Against this background of the current situation it is important to define the likely future needs and problems to try to define how solutions can be achieved.

The features to be determined

It has already been stressed that there is no clear definition of what we are trying to achieve when we undertake the current testing procedures or impose regulations based upon the results. The present overall concept is that we should aim at the reduction of the social and medical problems which are associated with drug **abuse**. No distinction is made between drug abuse in the socio-recreational scene or drug dependence in therapeutic use, yet there may be significant differences between these two problem areas, at least for some drug classes.

Moreover there is no conclusive evidence which shows that all the social problems among those who are either excessive users or abusers of drugs of dependence are caused specifically by the consumption of the drug. The use of the drug, whether this be legally or illegally procured, may itself be a response to social difficulties already encountered by the individual. It is therefore important to appreciate the nature of this relationship and take account of it when social problems are considered.

Licit or illicit abuse of many substances may give rise to social difficulties both within the narrow sphere of the group that directly surrounds the individual and in the wider sphere of the community at large. Changes of interpersonal relationships that stem from use of some of these drugs is an incontrovertible fact, but whether they are regarded as social problems depends on the views of the community, both small and large. This in its turn varies from one religion or ethos to another and, in the same community, from one generation to another. Consider, for example, the reaction of the community to the gin-sodden biddies of Hogarth cartoons, the laudanum takers of the Victorian era, the hashish users of the Middle East, opium smokers of China and psilocybin takers of the Central Americas. These substances have often been of considerable economic or social importance to the societies in which their use has been permitted or even encouraged. It is, in fact, often difficult to distinguish between accepted cultural use and abuse of the same drug in the community, because as social patterns of behaviour change, use can come to be regarded as abuse[6,8].

There is a need to define an unacceptable level of social disturbance that is produced by the drug, yet there are no finite standards on which it can be based. Until this can be done it is not possible to define the social aspects of the drug that need to be considered in the determination of the abuse and dependence risk.

The problem is even more difficult if we consider the existence of socially acceptable drugs of dependence such as alcohol and tobacco. There can now be no dispute that extensive social and medical costs follow the use of these substances. These include economic losses for the subject and his circle, deteriorating family and social relationships, and increased use of the social and medical services. To these social costs must also be added the public health costs of problems such as road traffic and industrial accidents, overdose deaths or morbidity, toxic psychoses and other mental and physical disorders not only for the individual but for those in the immediate neighbourhood. Yet despite clear evidence of dependence and of substantial social and public health cost (probably at least equal to those of some of the drugs which are controlled), no effective action is taken by authorities against these substances.

This must automatically call into doubt the whole current basis of present definitions of the substances of dependence and abuse that require attention on the grounds of social and medical costs. However great the difficulty that is involved action against all substances of abuse will only be logical when there are clear methods for the determination of the social and public health costs and action is taken in accordance with the findings that result.

Problems with new chemical classes

It is abundantly clear from what has been said already that while it is known that dependence risk always implies an action on the central nervous system there is no clear understanding of exactly what else leads to dependence or determines the level of risk of abuse. So far it appears that such diverse groups of substances as those acting on the chloride channel inhibitory mechanism, those acting as agonists or antagonists in the catecholamine reward areas, those acting on the endorphin-mediated pathways inter alia can all produce evidence of physical dependence on withdrawal. But within these classes the dependence risk does not always correlate with the abuse risk.

As has been stressed elsewhere in the book (Introduction) future research will lead to developments of chemical classes entirely different from those which currently exist. Some of these chemical classes or substances will, by accident or design, act on entirely different biochemical mechanisms within the central nervous system. We already know of numerous transmitter substances within the brain, and more transmitter mechanisms are being discovered each year. Yet we do not have any current understanding of which of these synaptic mechanisms have the characteristics that are susceptible to the generation of a dependence and abuse risk and which are not. If this is the situation for known chemical classes and known synaptic mechanisms, how much greater will be the difficulties in defining, in advance, the risks for new chemical classes acting on new synaptic mechanisms, unless the underlying principles can be established.

"Licit" analogues of illicit substances

Recent experience in the United States has demonstrated that those supplying the socio-recreational drug abuse scene may avoid the current regulations by the synthesis and supply of analogues of currently controlled substances which are not covered by the regulations. They do this without toxicity testing. This practice is particularly dangerous because some of these analogues have toxic effects which are not manifested by the parent compounds.

This raises the whole question of how far future legislation should cover substance classes rather than individual substances. Even more, within the current and future framework of a massive evil force based upon the profits of trading in drugs of abuse, it raises the question of how far governmental testing agencies should examine analogues of existing substances of socio-recreational abuse. The field is clearly enormous, and the cost implications disturbing.

Ethical considerations

The aim must remain the **prediction** of dependence and abuse risk before human exposure. This, however, is only possible if the preclinical methods have been adequately validated.

It has already been stressed that though there is broad validation for most of the current testing procedures these have not led to a determination of the underlying principles upon which it would be possible to base future predictions. Hence new preclinical methods will require human validation. This in its turn implies human experimentation.

Until relatively recently this human experimentation involved deliberate exposure to drugs of potential dependence risk, either with or without informed consent. Clearly studies without informed consent are ethically indefensible and cannot be used. There is greater difficulty over the ethical considerations surrounding such studies with so-called **informed** consent. Until the study is undertaken on a new substance or class the level and nature of the risk cannot be known, and hence the consent cannot be based on adequate information.

Yet coinciding with the sensible public debate about the validity of informed consent we have the consumer outcry for greater premarketing assured safety. These are, by their nature, mutually incompatible.

Studies on experimental animals

A recurring theme throughout the book is the demand of animal rights groups for at least a substantial reduction, and at best a total abolition, of experimentation on animals. Until there is an understanding of the basic mechanisms involved in the development of dependence and abuse, any substantial reduction in animal study is unlikely to be possible.

PATHWAYS TO FUTURE SOLUTIONS

It is abundantly clear from the foregoing that no current techniques exist for overcoming the anticipated needs and problems. If they did exist they would have been implemented already, for there are few, if any, who believe that our present techniques for the assessment of dependence and abuse risk are adequate. The future solutions must inevitably fall into two classes: pragmatic and fundamental.

Pragmatic future approach

Since a sine qua non of substance dependence is an effect on behavioural patterns via central nervous system activity, it follows that unless a substance produces effects within the central nervous system it will not produce dependence and/or abuse, at least by currently accepted mechanisms. Methods for animal testing for central nervous system behavioural effects are now well established. There will be the need, however, to make sure that these methods will apply to substances which act via different central nervous system mechanisms.

It follows that a logical method of screening for potential dependence and abuse will be a screen for central nervous system activity, updated as more reliable techniques are developed. Since abuse can occur not only to therapeutic substances but also to natural produces and household chemicals, it follows that all new substances should at least be subjected to a screen for central nervous system activity.

The second pragmatic approach stems from our present understanding of animal behavioural patterns during drug ingestion. As has been explained previously, while these methods have reasonable predictive value for substances that exert their effects by currently known mechanisms, they may have little or no relevance for new chemical classes.

Cross-substitution and withdrawal assessment studies in animals will require further refinement. In this respect it will be important for antagonists to be developed at an early stage in any such studies. These, by precipitating classical withdrawal reactions, should enable animal studies to be undertaken with fewer animals, at lower dose levels and after less extensive periods of administration[20].

Among more recent methods, perhaps the most encouraging group consists of self-administration techniques which assess the reinforcing properties of substances that are tested. It currently appears to provide valuable predictive information on the dependence risk of agonists, partial agonists and antagonists among the narcotic class; sedative compounds of alcohol, barbiturate and non-barbiturate hypnotic and tranquillizer type; compounds with psychomotor stimulant properties; volatile solvents and tobacco. These techniques do not, however, appear to demonstrate predictive value for the abuse of psychodelic substances. This is one specific indication that they may not be adequate for all future classes.

The interpretation of data from self-administration studies in animals is difficult because the effects depend upon such diverse effects as substance bioavailability, pharmacokinetics and direct behavioural effects. Attention has already been drawn to the possibility of rebound phenomena being confused with dependence withdrawal effects.

In order to improve their predictive value it is important for further basic work to be undertaken which will lead to further refinement of self-administration techniques. Self-administration may, for example, be encouraged by such extraneous factors as a sweet-flavoured solution by mouth in fluid-deprived animals. Such extraneous factors must be eliminated, as should pharmacological properties (e.g. sedation) which may influence the result. This will include such items as different routes of administration, the methods of intake reinforcement and the study of various primate and subprimatic species. The high cost of primate studies implies that validation of techniques for use in rodents and other less costly and less emotion-provoking species is a matter for urgent concern. Another important area for further research is the influence of the previous history of self-administration on the value of prediction for new substances. It may, for example, prove possible to sensitize animals to self-administer certain chemical classes by pretreatment. Despite the need to reduce animal studies, good prediction must for some time depend upon the appraisal of various animal techniques.

It will also be important to try to increase our understanding of the nature of the substance component of drug dependence and abuse, and hence to validate current predictive methods to derive general principles. This will involve such procedures as the correlation of self-administration studies in animals and man. Such studies should involve not only behavioural studies (e.g. psychometric tests, rating scales, questionnaires, etc.) but also classical physiological studies (e.g. biochemical, electrical, autonomic activity, etc.). Ethical problems associated with such studies have already been referred to, and will be considered in more detail later.

An important feature which requires urgent attention depends upon the difficulty in interrelating the results of different methods. This will involve consideration of "conceptual, methodological and empirical problems, including lack of comparability of studies . . ."[13].

Better human validation of animal data must be an important consideration despite the ethical problems that are involved.

Current studies involve mainly a cohort of hard-core abusers of multiple drugs. Future human studies should if possible involve in addition volunteers with various patterns of drug dependence and drug abuse. In these future studies it will be important to define methods for the assessment of more subtle behavioural effects (e.g. complex learning tasks, discrimination studies, problem solving). The studies should also examine the relationship between objective behavioural measurements (e.g. those operant procedures defined above) and the subjective rating of features of dependence.

The next area which requires a pragmatic approach, and

which must be solved if validation of animal studies is to be achieved, is increasing accuracy of adverse reaction recording.

Specific facilities for reporting, investigating and recording reputed adverse reactions have now been established by most national authorities. Doctors should be encouraged to report any suspected dependence to these units. In addition the manufacturer should be informed about such adverse reactions for most research-based pharmaceutical companies have full facilities for correlating the available data, and have a responsibility to determine the risk.

For any such assessment of the incidence of dependence under therapeutic conditions it is important to ensure that maximum information is recorded. The accuracy of the information should be independently cross-checked for each case as far as possible; those who are dependent are notoriously unreliable. Among information required is: the disorder that led to the administration of the drug; the age of the patient; previous use or abuse of drugs of potential dependence; current and previous levels of alcohol intake; the dose of the psychotropic prescribed; the dose of psychotropic actually taken; the length of administration.

Currently it is difficult to define withdrawal symptoms in objective terms, and objective measurements for these subjective phenomena should receive urgent consideration. This is rendered particularly necessary due to the fact that similar symptoms are common among normal people[21].

It is, however, not sufficient to record the cases but to attempt to express the incidence relative to the extent of usage. This can be based upon prescription audits, patient audits, manufacturers' figures and official statistics[6]. There is a measure of inaccuracy in each of these methods, and they have different sources of error. There are, therefore advantages in using several different measurements of usage to act as cross-checks.

Since one important feature of current socio-recreational abuse involves the use of multiple drugs[6] it is important that future animal pharmacological substitution and self-administration studies should involve drug interactions with classes of substances of known current abuse. For example one current, particularly unpleasant, abuse pattern involves the simultaneous intake of marijuana with "Mandrax", the synergistic effect of which in humans had not been predicted due to the lack of any animal studies.

One possibly important area of future research in animals which may have predictive value, but which may not be possible for emotional or ethical reasons, is the effect of drugs administered during pregnancy on the behavioural pattern of the offspring. Human experience suggests that the newborn are particularly susceptible to withdrawal.

Ultimately the "proof of the pudding must be in the eating", for there is no logical reason for predicting in advance that certain natural substances or general chemicals should be the subject of socio-recreational abuse (e.g. solvents). Hence a very important feature of abuse prevention must be a good reliable epidemiological survey of actual cases.

FUNDAMENTAL FUTURE APPROACHES

One important aspect of the future prediction of drug dependence and abuse is a better understanding of the relationship of drug-receptor interactions and their consequences to the substance component of the abuse phenomenon.

Currently agonists, partial agonists and antagonists related to some substances of abuse have been developed. It is desirable that this approach be extended to other chemical classes including those where classical animal dependence studies are not feasible (e.g. phychodelics). This must be matched by fundamental work on the receptors that are involved.

As it becomes possible to undertake work of this type involving different chemical classes it will be important to study the pharmacokinetic and pharmacodynamic aspects of these substance-receptor interactions, and to relate these to the tissue bioavailability and animal and human determination of abuse risk. If we are then to obtain a clearer understanding of the biological determinants of dependence and abuse we must extend such studies to the investigation of the central and peripheral biochemical changes to which these lead.

The movement away from the pragmatic and essentially haphazard approach to risk determination ultimately depends on a better understanding of the fundamental processes that are involved.

PHILOSOPHICAL CONSIDERATIONS

Attention has already been drawn to the ethical problems that exist over experimental animal and human study procedures. No less in the field of dependence than in any of the other areas of toxicity testing it is necessary for international legal, moral and scientific bodies to face up to the consideration of these ethical problems. Once an agreed formula has been reached it will be necessary for the leaders in society to encourage acceptance of the principles agreed.

The current conflict between the demands of society for protection against the risks of dependence, the political aspects of some international legislation, and the outcry of animal rights activists does little to stimulate internationally integrated investigation of this difficult subject.

Another area which requires philosophical consideration concerns the whole aspect of "pleasure-seeking behaviours"[6,17]. I have suggested in previous publications that such pleasure-seeking behaviour covers a broad spectrum ranging at one end from the narcotic abuse condemned by all to minor idiosyncrasies accepted by all as harmless[6,8]. The difficulty lies in establishing where in the central zone of the spectrum public health is at risk and protective action is required. Decisions about these matters are often based on political and economic expediency rather than a valid appraisal of the medical and social implications (e.g. alcohol, tobacco). There is an urgent need for a careful appraisal of the relative social cost of these pleasure-seeking behaviours. Social cost theory has now reached a stage at which such an appraisal is possible. For example, do the social costs of gambling represent a greater threat to society than the social costs of alcoholism; does the social benefit of tobacco in terms of employment and taxation outweigh its social and medical costs?

A similar matter of concern is the question of the cost-benefit of current legislative controls related to the level of dependence and abuse risk. There is still little evidence that drug abuse can be solved by legislation, yet legislation backed by police action is spreading into an ever-widening area of substance abuse without any consideration of cost-benefit appraisal. Perhaps the lead in suggesting a more realistic approach should be taken by toxicologists, who provide the basic data.

It does not seem logical that society should demand greater protection by means of more extensive toxicological study if it is not prepared to act rationally on the information that is already available on the social psychotropics.

I would also argue that the philosophical considerations go deeper than this, for we must also try to evaluate the worth of the toxicological information that is achieved against the extent of animal suffering, and decide by rational argument rather than emotion the level of animal study that can be justified.

CONCLUSIONS

By the use of the currently available techniques, and by developments that can be made, it should be possible to define the risk of dependence for substance classes that are currently known. Whether this will determine the abuse risk is a matter of dispute. Other substance classes, working by different mechanisms, will almost certainly be developed and will not be picked up by toxicological studies. Hence adverse reaction monitoring and epidemiological surveys should be an important aspect of strategic planning in this area.

However this does not take account of the philosophical considerations relating to society's approach to the management of the dependence and abuse problems.

REFERENCES

1. Eddy, NB, Halbach, H, Isbell, H and Seevers, MH (1965). Drug dependence: its significance and characteristics. Bull.WHO, 37, 1-12
2. WHO Expert Committee on Drugs Liable to Produce Addiction (1950). Report on the 2nd Session. World Health Org Tech Rep Ser No 21, Geneva
3. WHO Expert Committee on Drug Dependence (1969). Sixteenth Report. World Health Org Tech Rep Ser No 407, Geneva
4. Single Convention on Narcotic Drugs (1961). (New York: United Nations)
5. Convention on Psychotropic Substances (1971). (New York: United Nations)

6. Marks, J (1985). The Benzodiazepines: Use, Overuse, Misuse, Abuse?, 2nd edn. (Lancaster: MTP Press)
7. Lupolover, R, Dazzi, H and Ward, J (1982). Rebound phenomena: results of a 10 years' (1970-1980) literature review, Int Pharmacopsychiat, 17, 194-237
8. Glatt, MM and Marks, J (eds) The Dependence Phenomenon. (Lancaster: MTP Press)
9. Navaratnam, V (1982). Impact of scheduling drugs under the 1971 convention on psychotropic substances - the benzodiazepines reappraised, United Nations Research and Training Centre in Drug Dependence, National Drug Research Centre, Univ Science Malaysia, Minden, Penang, Malaysia
10. Edwards, G (1967). Personality and addiction. Howard J Penal Ref, 12, 136-9
11. WHO Expert Committee on Drug Dependence (1978). Twenty first Report. World Health Org Tech Rep Ser No 618, Geneva
12. WHO Expert Committee on Drugs Liable to Produce Addiction (1964). Report on the 13th Session. World Health Org Tech Rep Ser No 273, Geneva
13. Evaluation of dependence liability and dependence potential of drugs (1975). Report of a WHO Scientific Group. World Health Org Tech Rep Series No 577, Geneva
14. Fabre, LF, McLendon, DM and Harris, RT (1976). Preference studies of triazolam with standard hypnotics in out-patients with insomnia. J Int Med Res, 4, 247-54
15. Berger, H (1972). There are no addictive drugs, only addictive people. Postgrad Med, 51, 269-70
16. Keilholz, P (1971). Definition und Atiologe der Drogenabhangkeit, Bull Schweiz Akad Wiss, 27, 7-14
17. Keup, W (1982). Pleasure seeking and the aetiology of drug dependence, In Glatt, MM and Marks, J (eds). The Dependence Phenomenon. pp. 1-20. (Lancaster: MTP Press)
18. Thompson, T and Unna, KR (eds) (1977). Predicting the Abuse Dependence of Stimulant and Depressant Drugs. (Baltimore: University Park Press)
19. Silverman, PB and Ho, BT (1977). Characterization of discriminative response control by psychomotor stimulants. In Lal, H (ed.) Discriminative Stimulus Properties of Drugs. p. 107. (New York: Plenum Press)
20. Haefely, W, Polc, P, Pieri, L, Schaffner, R and Laurent, J-P (1983). Neuro-pharmacology of benzodiazepines: synaptic mechanisms and neural basis of action. In Costa, E (ed.), The Benzodiazepines: From Molecular Biology to Clinical Practice. pp. 21-66. (New York: Raven Press)
21. Merz, WA and Ballmer, U (1983). Symptoms of the barbiturate/benzodiazepine withdrawal syndrome in healthy volunteers: standardized assessment by a newly developed self-rating scale. J Psychoactive Drugs, 15, 71-84

PART 3
Preclinical:
In Vitro and *Ex Vivo* Approaches

12

Cellular and *In Vitro* Techniques

P. KNOX

This chapter will consider the attempts that have been made to date to make use of cells in culture to measure toxicity. The past decade has seen some major advances in biotechnology. For some years now it has been possible to isolate individual mammalian genes and to transfer these into bacteria, or indeed to other mammalian cells. By the construction of suitable sequences of DNA which contain promoting sequences as well as the gene in question, it is possible to achieve expression of the gene in an alien environment.

Advances have also taken place in other areas, and the production of monoclonal antibodies has revolutionized many areas of research and diagnosis.

At a time when it is relatively commonplace for laboratories to carry out one or more of the above techniques it is puzzling that so little biotechnological expertise has been applied to the area of toxicology and predictive safety evaluation. In this chapter, after a summary of cell culture techniques that have been applied to predictive safety evaluation, the technological innovations that should and probably will be made will be described. (Only a small number of typical references will be cited.)

CYTOTOXICOLOGY USING CELL CULTURES

Some definitions and descriptions may be useful at this stage for those readers who are not versed in the terminology of cell culture.

Cell cultures can be divided into three categories. Primary cultures are those derived directly from the tissues of animals or human beings. Cultures can be initiated by dissociating tissue or by allowing cells to migrate out of an explant. Cells will proliferate, and one advantage of either approach is that the cells are unlikely to have deviated significantly from their condition in vivo.

When the cells cease dividing, usually because of constraints of space within the culture vessel, the cells can be "subcultured"

171

into a number of fresh vessels. Cells will begin to proliferate and ultimately cover the new vessels. This process can be continued and the term "cell strain" is used to denote cells that have only gone through a limited number of divisions. Most cell strains can only be subcultured thirty or forty times before they begin to show signs of senescence. This process will be described in more detail later. Cells are no longer useful once the process of senescence has begun.

Some - a very small number - of cultures escape the senescence process and are said to be immortalized in that they can be subcultured almost indefinitely. These cells are then referred to as a cell line.

The advantages of cell lines are that homogeneous populations of cells can be maintained over lengthy periods of time. It is also true that the cell culture techniques involved are very much more simple.

The disadvantage of cell lines is that they can no longer be considered representative of a physiological system. Even at the chromosomal level cell lines are never diploid and many biochemical changes have taken place.

Established lines of cells are relatively easy to culture and stocks of cells are always available. BHK (baby hamster kidney) cells, for instance, were first derived in 1962 and various subclones have been used ever since. Despite the fact that the word kidney appears in the name, the cells are fibroblastic and derived from the connective tissue of the kidney rather than the parenchyma.

CHO (Chinese hamster ovary) cells are a line that has been much used. Again despite the name, the precise cellular origin of the cells is unknown. HeLa cells are a line that was not derived from normal tissue but rather from a cervical carcinoma.

The majority of the cell types that have been used in cytotoxicity assays have been fibroblastic. The reason for this is that fibroblasts are without doubt the simplest cell type to culture, and indeed the various aspects of cell culture methodology have been tailored to the growth of fibroblasts. This is clearly a problem as it is necessary to establish whether this is relevant to toxicity in vivo since connective tissue is not normally the target.

The end-points that have been used to measure toxicity are also numerous. Cell viability is one end-point that has been used; this can be judged by morphology or dye exclusion[1-3]. Measurement of cell growth has also been used; this method makes the assumption that a cell that has been affected by a toxic chemical will not be able to proliferate at optimal rates. Cell growth has been measured in a number of different ways. Cell number[4,5], total protein[6,7], protein synthesis and nucleic acid synthesis[8,9] are all parameters of growth and division. Finally release of intracellular components has also been extensively used; in particular, the release of enzymes since the assay of these is usually more sensitive[10,11].

As indicated, most studies have made use of cell lines that are usually said to be undifferentiated. A smaller number of studies have been reported which have made use of specialized cell types which maintain differentiated function in vitro.

The most frequent of these is the hepatocyte[12,13]. By cannulating the rat liver and perfusing with the enzyme collagenase it is possible to obtain a cell suspension of hepatocytes that retain many of their tissue-specific functions. Hepatocytes do not readily divide in vitro but will survive long enough to carry out assays of cytotoxicity. However it should be pointed out that, since cells do not survive in the long term, assays are carried out against a background of cell death. Far fewer studies have been carried out on epithelial cells from lung and kidney. In the case of lung toxicity, attention has been focused recently on pulmonary macrophages[14]. The logic for this step is that many compounds are converted to toxic products by the reticuloendothelial cells of the lung.

With the exception of genotoxicity and some aspects of neurotoxicity there is little in vitro toxicity testing that is carried out routinely. The research literature contains a large number of reports that conclude that in vitro methods could and should be used. While in most cases the accuracy of the experimental data cannot be questioned, the contribution of this literature to the future of in vitro toxicology testing is limited. This is due to a number of factors. Firstly, few attempts have been made to standardize the methodologies involved. Different cell types are often used and even when the same cell type is used the authors have utilized a different method of assay. Few independent reports have made use of the same toxic compounds, and only now are blind trials being carried out. These differences in technique make it impossible to evaluate reliability and reproducibility.

It must be stressed that there are a large number of variable parameters in cell culture, even for the growth of a given cell type. The growth medium consists predominantly of a chemically defined solution containing amino acids, vitamins, salts and a buffer system. There are many different formulations. In addition there has to be a supplement of plasma proteins, normally provided in the form of animal serum. This latter supplies proteins such as transferrin, albumin and a range of regulatory growth peptides which are all essential for cell survival and proliferation.

The different formulations of media and sera are bewildering and of great relevance to cytotoxicology testing since agents in the growth medium can modulate toxicity. Clearly it is necessary to achieve some degree of standardization, if only to be able to compare experimental data.

What is needed for cytotoxicological evaluation is a growth medium that is more representative of the conditions that cells will encounter in vivo. In the main, cell culture protocols have been devised to achieve maximal rates of cell growth. This often results in conditions that are very unphysiological.

As an example, sulphydryl containing amino acids can have a protective role against many toxic compounds since they influence levels of intracellular glutathione. Any agent which can modify cytotoxicity should be present in the growth medium in physiologically relevant concentrations.

Another deficiency in most of the experimental data is the failure to express the results in terms of in vivo toxicity. Results of such studies are normally expressed in terms of the concentration of a compound in the growth medium which brings about a 50% reduction in viability or in rates of proliferation. What is not currently established is how these values pertain to the toxicity in the whole animal or in man. This really is very important. Predictive safety evaluation requires a "no-effect" level and what is at present completely unknown is how to relate in vitro toxicity data with no-effect levels in vivo. Thus, despite assertions frequently made in the experimental literature, we are not yet at the stage when in vitro cytotoxicological data can be used. This will first require a large number of compounds to be evaluated in order to make the relevant correlations.

One large multicentre trial is now under way[15] and so far the results are promising. The trial has established that cell culture methods can be carried out reliably and reproducibly in different laboratories. A large number of coded chemicals is being tested in the presence and absence of a rat liver microsomal activating system. When all the compounds have been tested the code will be broken, and a correlation between in vitro and in vivo toxicity will be made. This will be the first time such an exercise has been carried out, thus highlighting the problem that, despite the large amount of purely experimental data, no experience has yet been gained as to reliability. Before one could countenance the possibility of replacing animal tests with in vitro assays the latter have to have proven reliability.

It is pertinent here to mention the consideration that went with the design of the protocol, since there are some requirements that will be the same for different areas of in vitro testing. The first is that the methods have to be as rapid and simple as possible without sacrificing accuracy. The number of compounds that require testing is very large and will presumably become even greater over the years. It is not practicable to have tests that are complex and require large numbers of highly trained personnel. Although it will be necessary to have some experienced workers, it will not be satisfactory if individuals require, say, 5 years training before they can carry out the basic techniques.

Expression of the results was also carefully considered. Obviously a numerical output is preferable since it makes it far simpler to categorize the toxicity of a compound. Morphological criteria are difficult to standardize and impossible to record in a simple fashion. They frequently need an expert simply to translate the original report.

There are some obvious advantages to the use of cell cultures. Some result from the fact that large numbers of replicate cultures can be established using multi-well tissue culture dishes. It is perfectly feasible for a single worker to manipulate many hundreds of such replicate cultures, and this enables dose-response relationships for a number of chemicals or pharmaceuticals to be obtained simultaneously. The reproducibility that is achieved is usually excellent.

An allied advantage is cost. The cost of production and use of a single well is less than one-hundredth that of the cost of single rodent. Clearly cost is a parameter that must be considered in the future of predictive safety evaluation. It is true that current conventional toxicology testing has and continues to identify compounds that have associated with them an unacceptable risk in terms of human exposure. What cannot be evaluated is how many chemicals and pharmaceuticals have their development discontinued because of unsuitable toxicological reports but would have posed no serious risk to man. There are a number of examples of pharmaceuticals that have been used for many years but would not today be taken onto clinical trials because of adverse results early during toxicological evaluation. Isoniazid is a good example to quote, since it has been used for more than two decades as an antitubercular drug but today would probably fail to complete a toxicological evaluation due to its toxicity in rats. This highlights the problem of interspecies variation; a compound that is highly toxic in an experimental animal may not necessarily be that toxic in man, and in any case risk assessment must include some consideration of benefit.

The problem of interspecies variation also highlights another advantage of cell culture; namely that it is possible to use cells of human origin. This is clearly most pertinent in the case of agents that are metabolized since most of the inter-species variation results from the different metabolic fate of chemicals in different animals.

The rest of the chapter will concern the developments that will occur between now and the end of the century. One of the factors that will change radically the methods used in cytotoxicology will be the use of novel biotechnological procedures in order to create vehicles designed specifically for predictive safety evaluation. In a nutshell, we should over the next decade aim to produce, by genetic manipulation, stable cell phenotypes that, by combining various tissue-specific functions, would enable many aspects of acute, chronic and target organ toxicity to be evaluated, using one or a limited number of cell types.

Molecular biology has developed so explosively that the number of individuals with experience in the techniques is very much smaller than the number of applications to which those techniques can be put. Both in industry and in academia there is a dearth of suitably trained scientists specializing in molecular biology, and thus one of the rate-limiting steps in the development of cytotoxicology will be the number of such competent personnel who apply themselves to the discipline.

There are many areas of research and development which can now be carried out using new molecular biological techniques. Many of these will have more rapidly realized gains, both financial and academic, than the development of vehicles for predictive safety evaluation. For instance, the financial gains of cloning one of the interferon genes are obvious, and would be realized in the short term. In contrast the advantages of a genetically engineered vector for toxicological evaluation would require greater vision.

As indicated earlier, the greatest problem appears to be the fact that many cell types do not express drug-metabolizing systems. The cells that do, in particular hepatocytes, although not difficult to obtain, suffer from several drawbacks. Reproducibility is not very good and cells can only be maintained for short time intervals. The end-points are also poorly defined. Similarly, microsomal fractions derived from liver are also variable, difficult to handle and have to be of animal origin. It is unlikely that human liver will ever be used in routine toxicology.

What is required is the production of a stable cell type that can be continuously cultured, is easy to manipulate and will express human drug-metabolizing systems. My laboratory, and hopefully others, are presently engaged in the development of such cell lines and the following approaches are being used.

In order to explain the approach that is being adopted we have to return to the subject of cell immortalization. It has been known for a number of years that cells both in vitro and in vivo exhibit programmed senescence. This is easy to observe in vitro since if primary cultures are set up from human tissues then the cells will go through a predictable number of cell divisions before senescence and finally cell death occurs. This process has been equated with natural ageing.

Some cells acquire genetic changes which enable them to escape this process. Activation of oncogenes is one mechanism whereby cells become immortalized. One oncogene that can be involved is the c-myc gene[16]. This gene encodes for a protein that is essential in the early phases of the cell proliferation cycle. If non-limiting amounts of the gene are transcribed and translated, cell division proceeds in an unrestricted fashion.

There are several ways in which this state of affairs can be brought about. The way it occurs naturally is probably through mutation or gene rearrangement such that uncontrolled levels of the protein for which it codes are produced. In the laboratory the gene and a promoter can be transfected directly into a given cell type.

Thus by transfecting suitable immortalizing oncogenes into specialized cell types which we have put into primary culture or have come from human neoplasms we hope to obtain a bank of cells which are stable and express the requisite cellular and biochemical functions.

Another approach that we are adopting is cloning the genes for human drug-metabolizing enzymes and transfecting these into suitable cellular vectors.

Bacterial genotoxicity testing is perhaps the only example where developments in cell and molecular biology have been put to use in predictive safety evaluation. The initial assumption is that a compound that is mutagenic in bacteria is likely to be a potential carcinogenic hazard in man. The tests make use of specific genetically selected bacterial strains and the methodology is described elsewhere in this volume. It is thus possible to carry out a rapid screen for agents that are able to induce point and frame-shift mutations.

However, this in vitro test using bacteria has its limitations, and there are many examples of carcinogens that do not prove to be mutagenic in bacteria. This is bound to be the case since some agents that are known to be carcinogenic interact with specific receptors. If bacteria do not synthesize the relevant receptor, there will be no effect in the in vitro assay. The cases when a bacterial system will be accurate are limited to those compounds that interact directly with the DNA. Some toxicologists do not routinely carry out bacterial genotoxicity testing as a primary screen, since it is felt that too many false negatives are obtained, for the reasons outlined here.

The other reason why the bacterial systems are limited is the complex aetiology of human tumours. Tumours do not arise as a result of single step but rather as the result of number of discrete steps. This multifactorial aetiology is obvious from epidemiological data and helps in part to explain the lengthy latent periods that are known to occur in human tumour induction. Long-term carcinogen testing is still necessary in predictive evaluation[17]. The reason is simply that any agent that increases the rate of occurrence of any of the events in the multifactorial pathway will increase tumour incidence. Certainly, carcinogen testing is fraught with difficulties, not the least of these being the high backgrounds of incidence found in experimental animals which probably result from unusual dietary regimes and a resulting abnormal endocrine status. However the testing is clearly reasonably effective.

What has hampered the development of better in vitro tests is the lack of knowledge of the carcinogenic mechanism. As indicated above it is far too simplistic to imagine that a single mutation can result in a tumour.

The past few years have seen a staggering output from molecular biology laboratories concerning the genetic and other changes that are involved in oncogenesis; in particular, the knowledge that all our cells contain proto-oncogenes, and that inappropriate expression of these is involved in the oncogenic event[18].

There are discrete classes of oncogenes. One of these is the class of oncogene that when activated brings about immortalization; these have been mentioned earlier. However when a cell is immortalized it will not form a tumour and another oncogene has to be activated for this transformation stage[19]. Many transforming oncogenes have now been identified. One that has attracted much attention is the psis gene[20] which has now been associated with a number of human tumours. Again the activation of the oncogene can be brought about by different mechanisms.

Many readers will be aware that oncogenes are often derived from viruses experimentally, and this often results in confusion since it is assumed that viruses are involved in the oncogenic activation. This is not the case, and indeed it is well established that viruses play little role in the majority of human tumours. However, experimentally, some viruses can be shown to be carcinogenic and this is because, during their life cycle inside a vertebrate host, viruses often incorporate regions of host DNA into the viral genome. Sometimes this DNA includes human proto-oncogenes. Now, if this becomes associated with a viral promoter region then, when a cell is reinfected with the virus, a segment of DNA can be reinserted into the host genome. The effect of the viral promoter is to bring about uncontrolled expression of the protein which was encoded by the gene originally picked up by the virus.

For a cancer to form, both immortalization and transformation have to occur. Another event that must occur is the stimulation of proliferation, since until the cell begins to divide it will not express its altered phenotype. A number of agents that do increase tumour incidence are effective because they stimulate inappropriate cell proliferation. If the affected cell goes on to form a tumour then genetic changes were already present in the cell. The situation is analogous to inducer/promoter experiments. In this latter case, high levels of the inducer that are used bring about both immortalization and transformation with the same agent. Clearly as the dose of a mutagen is increased the amount of affected DNA is greater, and this increases the chance that two different proto-oncogenes will become altered.

Thus the known multifactorial aetiology makes sense in that immortalization, transformation and growth stimulation are at least three events that have to occur.

This knowledge is important in the study of predictive safety evaluation since an insight into the various stages of oncogenesis can be detected by an effect on the cellular oncogenes themselves. The synthesis of the protein encoded by the oncogene might be studied, but almost certainly more suitable would be the use of a genetic probe to look directly at the DNA. While this latter sounds difficult this is not so. The techniques of molecular biology have been so refined over the past few years that it is now possible to screen for some inherited diseases using a complementary DNA (cDNA) sequence to probe the DNA extracted from a small number of cells taken from the fetus. In a similar fashion it will be possible to take human cells, expose them to test chemicals and then to use gene probes to see if oncogenes have been activated.

A word of caution has to be introduced, since it is not yet established as to how many oncogenes are involved in human tumours and whether a particular tumour type is associated with one or more different oncogenes. However, research in this area is progressing at such a rate that, by the end of the decade, it can be expected that most if not all oncogenic changes in human cells will have been characterized.

A complete knowledge of the mechanism and oncogenes involved in human tumours may not be necessary. Any agent that can bring about activation and expression of an oncogene in human cells must be considered a potential carcinogenic hazard.

In conclusion, while current attempts to use or validate in vitro methods is undoubtedly a necessary exercise, there will be severe limitations on their usefulness in predictive safety evaluation. However it is probably not exaggerating to predict that before the turn of the century it will be possible to construct a cell containing any combination of required genes. It should thus be possible to create vehicles expressing tissue-specific functions that could be used to measure different aspects of toxicology. It should even be possible to make many of these vehicles "self-indicating" in that by the insertion of particular gene functions at the relevant location, exogenous dyes would be altered when nearby genes are activated or when the cell is affected by a toxic agent. Similar procedures have already proved possible in the production of monoclonal antibodies.

REFERENCES

1. Inmon, J, Stead, A, Waters, MD and Lewtas, J (1981). Development of a toxicity test system using primary rat liver cells. In Vitro, 17, 1004-10
2. Scaife, MC (1982). An investigation of detergent action on cells in vitro and possible correlation with in vivo data. Int J Cosmetic Sci, 4 179-93
3. Kemp, RB, Meredith, RWS, Gamble, S and Frost, M (1983). Toxicity of detergent-based commercial products on cells of a mouse line in suspension culture as a possible screed for the Draize rabbit eye irritation test. ATLA, 11, 15-21
4. Ferguson, TFM and Prottey, C (1974). A simple and rapid method for assaying cytotoxicity. Food Cosmet Toxicol, 14, 431-4
5. Litwin, J, Enzell, C and Pilotti, A (1978). The effect of tobacco smoke condensate on the growth and longevity of human diploid fibroblasts. Acta Pathol Microbiol Scand, 86, 135-41
6. Valentine, R, Chang, MJW, Hart, RW, Finch, GL and Fisher, GL (1983). Thermal modification of chrysotile asbestos: evidence for decreased cytotoxicity. Envir Health Perspect, 51, 357-68
7. Williams, GM (1974). The direct toxicity of alpha-naphthylisothiocyanate in cell culture. Chem Biol Interact, 8, 363-9
8. Cheng, Y-C, Derse, D, Tan, RS, Dutschman, G, Bobek, M, Schroeder, A and Bloch, A (1981). Biological and biochemical effects of 2'-azido-2'-deoxyarabinofuranosylcytosine on human tumor cells in vitro. Cancer Res, 41, 3144-9
9. Pawlak, K, Matuszkiewicz, A, Pawlak, JW and Konopa, P (1983). The mode of action of cytotoxic and antitumor 1-nitro-acridines. Chem Biol Interact
10. Abernathy, CO, Lukacs, L and Zimmerman, HJ (1975). Toxicity of tricyclic antidepressants to isolated rat hepatocytes. Biochem Pharmacol, 24, 347-50
11. Tyson, CA, Mitoma, C and Kalivoda, J (1983). Evaluation of hepatocytes isolated by a nonperfusion technique in a prescreed for cytotoxicity. J Toxicol Envir Health, 6, 197-205
12. Casini, AF and Farber, JL (1981). Dependence of the carbon tetrachloride-induced death of cultured hepatocytes on the extracellular calcium concentration. Am J Pathol, 105, 138-48
13. McQueen, CA and Williams, GM (1982). Cytotoxicity of xenobiotics in rat hepatocytes in primary culture. Fund Appl Toxicol, 2, 139-44
14. Bally, MB, Opheim, DJ and Shertzer, HG (1980). Di-(2-ethylhexyl) phthalate enhances the release of lysosomal enzymes from alveolar macrophages during phagocytosis. Toxicology, 18, 49-60
15. Balls, M and Bridges, JW (1983). The FRAME research programme on in vitro toxicology. In Goldberg, AM (ed.) Alternative methods in Toxicology. Vol 2, pp. 61-79. (New

York: Mary Ann Liebert)

16. Land, H, Parada, LF and Weinberg, RA (1983).   Tumorigenic conversion of primary mouse embryo fibroblasts requires at least two cooperating oncogenes.   Nature, 304, 596-602

17. Purchase, IFH (1982).   An appraisal of predictive tests for carcinogencity.   Mutat Res, 99, 53-71

18. Temin, HM (1984).   Do we understand the genetic mechanisms of oncogenesis? J Cell Physiol Suppl, 3, 1-11

19. Ruley, HE (1983).   Adenovirus early region 1A enables viral and cellular transforming genes to transform primary cells in culture.   Nature, Lond, 304, 602-6

20. Gazit, A, Igarashi, H, Chiu, I-M, Srinivasan, A, Yaniv, A, Tronik, SR, Robbins, KC and Aaronson, SA (1984).   Expression of the normal human sis/PDGF-2 coding sequence induces cellular transformation.   Cell, 39, 89-97

13
Immunological Aspects

K. MILLER AND S. NICKLIN

GENERAL CONCEPTS OF THE IMMUNE SYSTEM

In order to survive and resist invasion by parasitic and pathogenic
micro-organisms, multicellular life forms evolved a variety of
specific and non-specific defence mechanisms. The present-day
vertebrate immune system therefore represents the end-result of a
series of gradual adaptive cellular and chemical responses designed
to ensure the survival of a species in the face of a changing and
potentially hostile environment. Our understanding of immunity and
the immune system as a whole has, over the past few decades, ma-
tured rapidly from the early recognition of non-specific or natural
resistance to infectious agents - mediated for example by complement and lysozymal enzymes. This evolved to an appreciation of
distinct specific cell-mediated and humoral responses, and more
recently the identification and functional characterization of various
subpopulations of lymphoid cells[1]. Analysis of immune responses
in man and experimental animals has revealed the immune system to
be a finely tuned and precisely controlled mechanism involving multiple integrated reactions between subsets of thymus-matured lymphocytes (T cells), bone marrow/bursa-matured lymphocytes (B
cells) and a variety of antigen-processing and accessory cells of
macrophage origin. These cells interact either directly or indirectly
with a battery of other cell types including natural killer cells,
eosinophils, and mast cells. Cell-cell communications have been
shown to occur by direct cell contacts or via the release of cell
products either into the cellular microenvironment or systematically
into the circulation. These secreted cell products include the prostaglandin and leukotriene variety of as yet undefined immunoreac-
tive molecules[2-4]. This facility for cell-to-cell communication
provides a complex homeostatic mechanism which can both direct
and regulate the immune reaction. In addition to this network of
intercellular communication the integrity of the system may be further modified by the endocrine/neurological axis as well as by
nutritional or environmental factors[5].

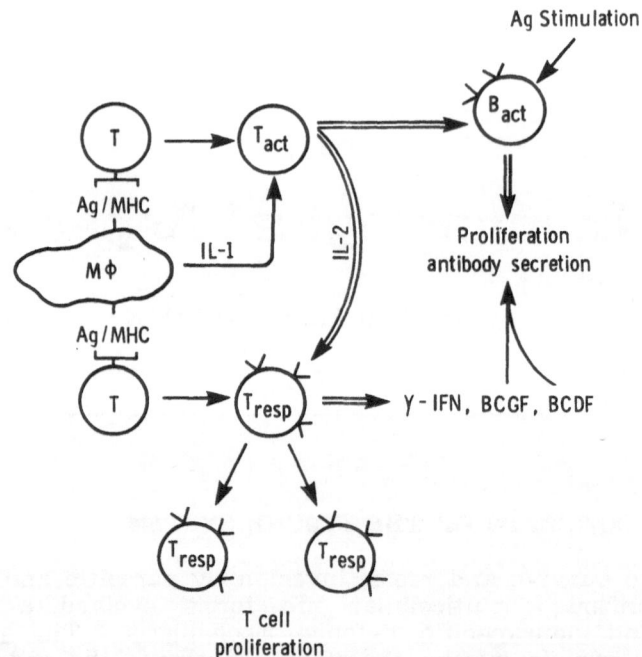

Figure 13.1   Clonal expansion of T lymphocytes after antigen presentation. T_{act} = activated T lymphocyte; T_{resp} = responder population; B_{act} = activated B lymphocyte; Ag/MGC = antigen and major histocompatibility receptors; IL1 = interleukin 1; IL-2 = interleukin 2; gamma-IFN = gamma interferon; BCGF = B cell growth factor; BCDF = B cell differentiation factor

Under normal circumstances when antigen-reactive cells of the immune system are confronted by antigen a complex, interrelated sequence of genetically preprogrammed, histocompatibility-restricted events are initiated. The macrophage is usually the first cell to encounter antigen; it phagocytoses, digests and processes the material prior to presenting antigenic components to antigen receptive T cells. As a consequence the T cells are triggered to undergo clonal expansion (Figure 13.1). Subgroups of antigen-reactive cells include those that function as regulatory cells (helper or suppressor T cells), those involved in cytotoxic reactions (Figure 13.2) and T lymphocytes involved in delayed-type hypersensitivity responses. During this phase of the reaction, antigen-primed T helper cells may interact with appropriate antigen receptive B cells and trigger the B cells to proliferate and differentiate into either plasma cells, which go on to secrete antibodies with specificity for the antigen, or a population of long-lived memory cells ready to respond in an anamnestic fashion on subsequent re-exposure to the antigen, (for general review see Refs. 1, and 6-8).

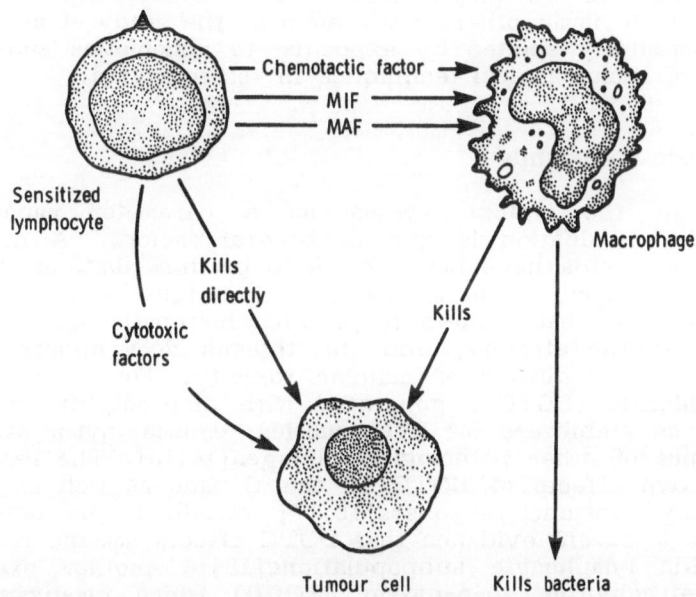

Figure 13.2 Activation of cytoxic effector functions of T lymphocytes and macrophages. MIF = macrophage inhibitor factor;
MAF = macrophage activating factor

This co-operative cellular interaction between the components
of cellular and humoral immunity usually maintains an effective
mechanism for the defence of the host against invasion by viruses,
fungi, bacteria and parasites. It also provides a facility whereby
the host's own cells may be continually monitored for neoplastic
change (immunosurveillance). Indeed it has been postulated that
the failure of the immune system to recognize these mutant cells
plays a causal role in the development of tumours.

There are, however, circumstances when the immune system
does not always serve in the best interest of the host. Immune
mechanisms are, for example, responsible for the rejection of
potentially beneficial tissue transplants as well as the pathogenesis
of several disease processes including anaphylactic reactions, contact sensitivity, immune complex diseases and a variety of autoimmune disorders. Since immune responses to some extent function as
a double-edged sword, in the sense that they can be either beneficial or detrimental to the host, agents which interfere with the
normal functioning of the immune system must be treated with particular caution.

RELEVANCE OF IMMUNOLOGY IN SAFETY EVALUATION STUDIES

The main areas currently relevant to immunotoxicology have been
identified as the study of adverse immunological events associated

with exposure of man and animals to xenobiotics, exposure of man and animals to immunotherapeutic agents, the study of allergenicity and autoimmunity elicited by exposure to xenobiotics and the application of immunological techniques in toxicology[9].

Immunotoxic compounds

Interest in the immune system as a parameter important in toxicological evaluation is due to several factors. A number of diverse compounds have been shown to produce distinct effects on the immune competence of laboratory animals[10-13]. Many of these compounds have been shown to produce histopathological changes, including thymic atrophy, and the thymus does appear to be a very sensitive indicator of cellular toxicity. For example, di-n-octyl-dichloride (DOTC), generated with di-n-octyltin derivatives are used as stabilizers for PVC plastics, causes thymic atrophy in the absence of other pathological changes[14,15]. The reasons for the selective effects of DOTC on the thymus as well as on some cell-mediated immune responses[16,17] remain to be determined, but there is recent evidence that DOTC affects immune recognition by specific lymphocyte subpopulations[18]. Another example is 2,3,7,8-tetrachlorobenzo-p-dioxin (TCDD) which produces thymic atrophy at extremely low levels of exposure[19]. Available data indicate that the TCDD-induced thymic atrophy is due to a ligand-like interaction with a receptor, the Ah receptor[20]. Furthermore, there is experimental evidence that very low dose levels of TCDD cause alterations of the intrathymic environment, (mediated by the Ah receptor), which leads to the loss of cytotoxic T cell populations. These and similar experiments demonstrate the complexity of the immune system and focus attention on two important questions. Firstly, whether exposure to xenobiotics which alter the immune status can result in enhanced risk of specific diseases, and secondly, whether immune suppression may serve as a co-factor in chemically induced neoplasia.

A number of studies have demonstrated specific and non-specific immune responses against experimentally induced immunogenic tumours as well as enhanced growth of tumours and/or increased metastatic spread in immunologically depressed animals[21,22]. More importantly, from the toxicologist's point of view, an enhanced incidence of tumours induced by ultraviolet light, methylcholanthrene or benzo(alpha)pyrene has been demonstrated in mice treated with immunosuppressive agents[23,24]. Such data are consistent with the hypothesis that a correlation exists between the administration of chemical immunosuppressants and an increased incidence of certain types of neoplasia in laboratory animals.

Whilst there are inherent difficulties in the transfer of data from animal experimentation to man, it is equally difficult to select a population environmentally or occupationally exposed to compounds at levels which could alter immune regulatory mechanisms. Perhaps the most appropriate investigation relates to the incident in Michigan, USA, in 1973 when a preparation of polybrominated biphenyls (PBB) was accidentally mixed into cattle feed. As a consequence dairy products and meat containing PBB was widely consumed by the Michigan residents. A significant depression of cell-mediated immune responsiveness was demonstrated in this population[25,26] and preliminary reports have noted an increase in tumour incidence in individuals with confirmed immune dysfunction.

A special case may be made for asbestos-associated diseases. Silica and asbestos dusts have repeatedly been shown to have differing effects on the alveolar macrophage and its immunoregularity functions[27]. The lack of association between silicosis and the development of neoplasms, compared with that of asbestosis, has led immunotoxicologists to suggest that exposure to asbestos might induce an immune imbalance that renders the host more susceptible to the carcinogenic potential of asbestos fibres. Evidence acquired from studies of immunosuppressed patients and of those with acquired immune deficiencies has also been cited as an illustration of the harmful consequences that may occur after exposure to immunotoxic compounds. It was concluded at the Luxembourg Seminar (1984)[9], on the basis of both animal studies and clinical investigations, that harmful consequences to human health may derive from exposure to immunotoxic compounds, and that the development of methods that may be of value in immunotoxicological risk assessment be given priority status.

Biological response modifiers

The assessment of potential undesirable consequences of biological response modifiers (BRMs) and monoclonal antibodies, whose primary activity may be targeted on the immune system, has presented the immunotoxicologist with a special set of problems[28,29]. The effect of these therapeutic agents has been shown to be a multi-phase phenomenon; that is, administration of a compound leads to several phases of stimulation and depression over a comparatively small dose range[30]. There is no indication at present of what the mechanism of the effect might be. If the effector cells of the immune system, or the helper cells that control them, were divided into numerous subpopulations, with different thresholds of responsiveness to the BRMs, some might respond to low and intermediate doses of the agent, while others might be "switched-on" or alternatively "switched off". Another mechanism might involve the differential stimulation of different effector cell populations. For example, in studies on the effect of BCG vaccine on B6AF mice Davies and Sabbatini[31] found that the response could be mediated either by both T lymphocytes and macrophages or solely by T cells. As the dose may act as a continuous variable it is essential that dose-response relationships are firmly established and understood. Much research is still needed in this area.

Mechanisms are easier to analyse in vitro than in vivo, and the use of homogeneous cloned cell populations, rather than the complex mixtures of cell types and specificities found in lymphoid organs, could be a powerful aid in understanding the spectrum of immune effects inducible by BRMs. Such studies would in turn lead to more meaningful in vivo evaluations of the potential benefit of

BRMs and alleviate excessive deviation from normal immune function.

Autoimmunity

A number of drugs have been reported to cause symptoms associated with autoimmune phenomena in susceptible patients, and such a possibility should be taken into consideration during evaluations of safety with the formation of immune complexes and the development of autoimmune reactions monitored.

The development of autoimmune disease results from the breakdown of the normal homeostatic immunological regulatory mechanisms that prevent the stimulation of self-reactive lymphocytes. This reaction, in turn, leads to the expansion of autoreactive lymphocytes and autoantibodies, and all autoimmune reactions, whether humoral or cellular, are directed against autoantigens. Under certain conditions self-structures could also be rendered non-self by a foreign agent and an autoimmune reaction ensue. One recent experimental approach has been to link the induction of autoimmune phenomena with the graft-versus-host like reactions (GVHR) stimulated in autologous and syngeneic mice by drugs such as diphenyltoin[32]. The data are consistent with the concept that the drug, or its metabolites, can modify cell surface determinants in such a way that T lymphocytes respond in a manner comparable to the reactions of parental strain T cells to the allogeneic structures on F_1 recipient cells. It is advocated that this animal model could help in the elucidation of the genetic and cellular alterations needed for the development of GVHR-like lesions after sensitization by drugs or other aetiological agents.

Hypersensitivity reactions

The major clinical manifestations of chemically induced immunotoxicity are hypersensitivity (allergic) reactions. Numerous biological test procedures in man and in laboratory animals have been developed for studying the induction and elicitation phases of contact sensitivity, and data on the ability to induce contact sensitivity are required by regulatory authorities. In particular, a considerable amount of work has been done over the years to develop procedures for detecting sensitizing effects of chemicals on laboratory animals in order to preselect compounds unlikely to be well tolerated by man[33-35]. Although the majority of test procedures are accepted, there is an acknowledged need for improvement and standardization of techniques for the development and validation of in vitro models, and for better information on the minimal doses of chemicals required to induce or elicit hypersensitivity responses. The present consensus is that, in many cases, screening of chemicals by the usual testing procedures gives an adequate basis for use, but that questionable reactivity requires further investigation into mechanisms. It has recently been recommended that the screening of compounds to be marketed should include trials on human volunteers with particular reference to the vulnerability of certain groups, and that such studies should be undertaken in community health centres or their equivalent, prior to general release.

It must be emphasized that there is, at present, no suitable animal model for assessing the allergic potential of ingested or inhaled materials. There is a real need for the development of a model for these, in the main, antibody-mediated reactions, and for research to be carried out on the basic mechanisms concerned in adverse reactions to food additives and in the development of occupational asthma.

METHODOLOGY FOR TOXICOLOGICAL EVALUATION

As described earlier, the cellular interactions involved in immune responses are very complex, and their regulation and feedback control influenced by pharmacological mediators and a number of modifying host factors. In view of the complexities of such multifactorial influences the use of animal models is unavoidable in providing essential information, particularly with respect to the functional reserve of the immune system and its ability to recover from toxic insult. However, if one simply states that a compound affects the immune response, without defining the locus of action, a major opportunity in predicting the effects of future classes of xenobiotics could be missed. In areas such as these, in vitro assays could well give insights into the mechanism of action, as well as aid in designing meaningful predictive studies in the intact animal. Before discussing these future perspectives, however, it might be well to summarize the two approaches to immunotoxicological evaluation which are currently advocated.

One approach is that of the Dutch National Institute of Health, which is to undertake histopathology of the lymphoreticular system in subacute toxicity studies on random-bred Wistar rats[10]. Only if changes are seen at this stage would more specific immunological investigations be undertaken. There are obvious advantages in using animals from routine studies, but this immunopathological approach includes special techniques such as enzyme histochemistry, immunocytochemistry, and the enumeration of bone marrow stem-cell populations, techniques not normally included in evaluation of toxicity. In addition there is some evidence that such an approach may not be sufficiently sensitive at dose levels that do not cause discernible deterioration of general health, or where the effects on another organ may indirectly modulate the immune response[36,37].

The second approach is to generate data specifically relevant to immune functions during subacute toxicity testing, perhaps on a flexible tiered system. Experimental investigations currently in progress in the USA, under the National Toxicicology Program for Immunotoxicity Assessment, have included functional and host resistance assays as well as immunopathology in studies on B6C3F1 mice. Lymphocyte mitogen responses, one-way mixed leukocyte cultures, natural killer cell cytolysis, peritoneal macrophage function, antibody plaque-forming cells and PYB6 sarcoma and Listeria monocytogenes models for measuring host resistance are among the in vitro and in vivo methods being evaluated in order to find the tests that would give the optimal amount of information[5,38].

This approach, however, is compromised by questions concerning the functional immune reserve for each parameter measured, and thus its biological significance. Many minor changes in immune responsiveness occur daily under the influence of environmental pathogens or drugs without, for example, undue susceptibility to infection. On the other hand, even mild immunosuppression may be a potential danger in a vulnerable population group. The ideal assessment of immunotoxicity in the whole animal, perhaps utilizing a few selective assays in a sequential fashion, is still in evolution.

Nevertheless there is no doubt that in many cases information can be provided by novel and potentially useful in vitro models. Experimental approaches designed to investigate the molecular biology of cell-cell interactions and their products, and the effects of xenobiotics on both the genome and DNA repair mechanisms will undoubtedly find a place in the future immunotoxicological assessment regimens. Some of the more promising models with possible future applications are discussed in the following section.

IN VITRO MODELS

Binding studies

A good deal of toxicity may centre around interferences with the ability of cells to interact and communicate with each other. Some of these interactions are mediated by soluble factors such as immunoglobulins or interleukins, which can serve as chemical messengers that transmit information between widely separated cells. In other cases interactions require physical contact between cells, and cell-cell adhesion, and depend upon cell surface proteins such as histocompatibility antigens, immunoglobulin and interleukin receptors and the T-cell receptor. Indeed, much of what is currently known about immune responses has been discovered at the cellular level, through purification and cloning of the cells involved and through the use of molecular biology and monoclonal antibody technology to determine the structure and function of cell-surface proteins. This knowledge could usefully be employed for developing more sophisticated in vitro assays for evaluating whether compounds could influence immune reactions and to characterize those individual events that might lead to alterations in immune balance.

For example, macrophages play a primary role in both non-specific defence mechanisms and the initiation and regulation of immune responses, and the effect of particulate matter on macrophages has been studied in a number of in vitro and in vivo systems[39-41]. In general, peritoneal or alveolar macrophages have been obtained from laboratory animal models, although alveolar macrophages obtained from the lungs of cattle at slaughter have been utilized to evaluate the relative toxicity of trace metals and combustion products[42]. The bovine model has the advantage that large quantities of alveolar macrophages are harvested from one donor resulting in a genetic and historic homogeneity that may be lacking when alveolar macrophages from many donors are pooled. Macrophage-like cell lines such as P388D have also been utilized so as to enable assays to be performed under identical conditions on a homogeneous population. Until recently, available cell lines have been defective in one or more functions characteristic of untransformed macrophages. Now, however, human monocytes have been transformed into macrophage-like cell lines which express HLA-DR and DS determinants[43]. These antigen-presenting cell lines are able to stimulate a mixed lymphocyte reaction as well as possessing the expected characteristics of mononuclear phagocytes such as lysozyme secretion, phagocytosis and expression of Fc and complement receptors. They should provide a valuable model for evaluating the effect of compounds on several macrophage functions, including those directly pertinent to immune regulation.

The ability to clone single T cells is a most useful achievement because the progeny in any one clone will be of a single functional subtype and, at the very least, will have the great specificity associated with monoclonality. Such technology has been applied to studies of the receptors and products of T cells and their means of activation and regulation[44].

Functional human T-cell clones are now available in many laboratories and multiple monoclonal antibodies to their surface molecules exist. T-cell clones could therefore be used for investigating whether compounds interact with receptors on their membrane, particularly if a functional factor associated with that receptor expression could be measured. Interleukin 2 (IL-2), originally termed T-cell growth factor, represents one such factor, and release of IL-2 receptor-positive T cell, regardless of its subclass and antigenic specificity. All subclasses of T cells have been shown to release IL-2 under appropriate conditions although helper T cells appear to be the major source[45], and factors with IL-2 activity prepared from human, ape, rat and murine cells are all analogues of one another[46]. The activity of IL-2 present in the medium after administration of test compound to the chosen T lymphocyte clone is easily quantitated by using an IL-2-dependent cell line. The murine cytoxic T-cell line CTLL is widely used as the target cell and activity of IL-2 may be assayed by measuring the dilution limit at which the interleukin still exerts its growth-stimulating effect on the target cell. Should the test compound block IL-2 production then a further test to ascertain whether it could influence the immune response in vivo would be undertaken, or alternatively such an in vitro assay might give some insight as to whether compound modification should be considered.

Another area where binding studies could serve as markers for the possibility that compounds might interfere with the immune system is chemotaxis, the sequential process of receptor-mediated recognition and arrival of tissue-specific and antigen-specific lymphocytes of the appropriate specificities at sites of antigen accumulation. Receptors such as surface immunoglobulins, the antigen receptor or B lymphocytes[47], are distinguished by their capacity to stimulate chemotaxis, in vitro, chemotaxis to gradient concentration of anti-immunoglobulin can be shown directly in B lymphocytes[48]. Prior incubation with test compounds would there-fore be a measure of the ability of such compounds to block or in-terfere with an activity directly related to ligand interaction with the surface immunoglobulin receptor.

It is recognized that binding to a B cell, or a T cell or a macrophage, does not necessarily implicate that a compound is im-munotoxic, but following such initial observations appropriate im-munological function tests could be undertaken to evaluate the potential effect on immune responses.

DNA repair defects and immunodeficiency

Damage to DNA and its defective repair might be involved in deranged immune functions leading to deficiency and autoimmune states as well as lymphoid neoplasia.

Indeed, several human diseases associated with defective DNA repair show evidence of immunological defects[49]. One ex-ample is the description of a patient with severe immunodeficiency, whose fibroblasts were hypersensitive to a wide range of agents which damage DNA, suggesting the presence of DNA repair defects[49]. Another example is the in vitro studies of the repair of O6-methylguanine in human lymphocytes obtained from patients with various autoimmune diseases which were found unable to repair the lesion proficiently[50].

Mathematical models

In general, immunotoxicology is now at a stage where events are being characterized individually. These events are very complicated and involve many components, and no doubt theoretical models could be useful adjuncts to experimental work and screening assays[51]. Models could contribute to the design of experimental methods and interpretation of data. They might suggest when to take samples, which dose levels to use, and explore how cellular interactions in vivo could be quantitated and simulated. Such models could be deterministic, and consist of a series of equations which describe the immune phenomena mathematically, or they may be stochastic and consist of equations which would determine the probabilities of a particular event. In either method, a computer may be used to perform the numerical and stochastic analysis required to apply to the model to a given set of conditions.

CONCLUSIONS

At present the appropriate animal/in vitro models to assess the full range of possible immunological consequences that may occur in response to toxic insult are not readily available. New avenues of immunotoxicity testing must therefore be explored before it will be possible to develop tests with the capacity fully to evaluate new compounds in terms of their immunopharmacological and immuno-toxicological effects.

REFERENCES

1.   Miller, JFAP (1978). The cellular basis of immune responses. In Samter, M (ed.) Immunological Diseases, pp.35-48. (New York: Little Brown)
2.   Rumjanek, VM, Hanson, JM and Moreley, J (1982). Lymphokines and monokines. In Sirois, P and Rola-Pleszczynksi, M (eds.) Immunopharmacology, pp.267-86. (Amsterdam: Elsevier)
3.   Bloom, BR (1980). Interferons and the immune systems. Nature, 284, 593-5
4.   Nicklin, S and Shand, FL (1982). Abrogation of suppression cell function by inhibitors of prostaglandin synthesis. Int. J. Immunopharmacol., 4, 407-14
5.   Dean, JH, Luster, MI, Bourman, GA and Lauer, LD (1982). Procedures available to examine the immunotoxicity of chemicals and drugs. Pharmacol Rev, 34, 137-48
6.   Ohanve, ER (1972). The regulatory role of macrophages in antigenic stimulation. Adv Immunol, 15, 95-105
7.   Raff, MC and Cantor, H (1971). Subpopulations of thymus cells and thymus-derived lymphocytes. Prog Immunol, 1, 83-97
8.   Katz, DH and Benacerraf, B (1972). The regulatory influence of activated T cells on B cell responses to antigen. Adv Immunol, 15, 1-11
9.   International Seminar on the Immunological System as a Target for Toxic Damage, Luxembourg, 6-9 November 1984
10.   Vos, JG (1977). Immune suppression as related to toxicology. CRC Crit Rev Toxicol, 5, 67-101
11.   Koller, LD and Roan, JG (1980). Effects of lead, cadmium and methylmercury on immunological memory. J Environ Pathol Toxicol, 4, 47-52
12.   Faith, RE, Luster, MI and Vos, JG (1980). Effects on immune competence by chemicals of environmental concern. In Hodgson, E, Bend, JR and Philpot, RH (eds.) Reviews in Biochemical Toxicology, 2, pp.173-211 (Amsterdam: Elsevier)
13.   Miller, K (1985). Immunotoxicology. Clin Exp Immunol, 61, 219-23
14.   Seinen, W and Willens, MI (1976). Toxicity of organotin compounds. I. Atrophy of thymus and thymus-dependent lymphoid tissue in rats fed di-n-octyl tin dichloride. Toxicol Appl Pharmacol, 35, 63-75
15.   Miller, K, Scott, MP and Foster, JR (1984). Thymic involution in rats given diets containing dioctyltin dichloride. Clin Immunol Immunopathol, 30, 62-70
16.   Seinen, W, Vos, JG, van Krieken, R, Penninks, AH, Brands, R and Hooykaas, H (1977). Toxicity of organotin compounds. III. Suppression of thymus-dependent immunity in rats by di-n-butyltin dichloride and di-n-octyltin dichloride. Toxicol Appl Pharmacol, 42, 213-24
17.   Miller, K and Scott, MP (1985). Immunological consequences of dioctyltin dichloride (DOTC)-induced thymic injury. Toxicol Appl Pharmacol, 78, 395-403
18.   Miller, K, Maisey, J and Nicklin, S (1985). Effect of orally administered dioctyltin dichloride on murine immune com-

petence. Environ Res (In press)

19. Veichi, A, Sironi, M, Canegrati, MA, Recchia, M and Garattini, S (1983). Immunosuppressive effects of 2,3,7,8-tetrachlorodibenzo-p-dioxin in strains of mice with different susceptibility to induction of aryl hydrocarbon hydroxylase. Toxicol Appl Pharmacol, 68, 434-41

20. Lund, J, Kurl, RN, Pellinger, L and Gustaffson, JA (1982). Cytosolic and nuclear binding proteins for 2,3,7,8-tetrachlorodibenzo-p-dioxin in the rat thymus. Biochem Biophys Acta, 716, 16-23

21. Baldwin, RW (1983). Specific antitumor immunity and its role in host resistance to tumors. In Herberman, RB (ed.) Basic and Clinical Tumor Immunology, pp.107-128. (New York: Academic Press)

22. Frost, P and Kerbel, RS (1983). Immunology of metastasis: can the immune response cope with disseminated tumor? Cancer Metastasis Rev, 2, 239-56

23. Outzen, HC (1980). Development of carcinogens - induced skin tumors in mice with varied states of immune capacity. Int J Cancer, 260, 87-94

24. Kalland, T and Forsberg, JG (1981). Natural killer cell activity and tumor susceptibility in female mice treated neonatally with diethylstilbesterol. Cancer Res, 41, 5134-40

25. Bekesi, JG, Holland, JF, Anderson, HA, Fischbein, AS, Rom, W, Wolff, MS and Selikoff, IJ (1978). Lymphocyte function of Michigan dairy farmers exposed to polybromenated biphenyls. Science, 199, 1207-9

26. Bekesi, JF, Roboz, JP, Solomon, S, Fischbein, AD and Selikoff, IJ (1983). In Gibson, GG, Hubbard, R and Parke, DV (eds.) Immunotoxicology, pp.181-191 (London: Academic Press)

27. Miller, K (1979). Alterations in the surface-related phenomena of alveolar macrophages following inhalation of crocidolite asbestos and quartz dusts: an overview. Environ Res, 20, 162-82

28. Vitetta, ES and Uhr, JW (1984). The potential use of immunotoxins in transplantation, cancer therapy, and immunoregulation. Transplantation, 37, 535-8

29. Spreafico, F (1984). Immunomodulation by xenobiotics: the open field of immunotoxicology. In Fudenberg, HH, Whitten, HD and Ambrogi, F (eds.) Immunomodulation: New Frontiers and Advances, pp.311-330 (New York: Plenum Press)

30. Davies, M (1983). Phase variations in the modulation of the immune response. Immunol Today, 4, 103-6

31. Davies, M and Sabbatini, E (1978). Effect of BCG on alloimmune cell-mediated cytotoxicity in (C57BL/6J female XA/J male) F1 mice. J Natl Cancer Inst, 60, 1059-73

32. Gleichmann, E, Pals, ST, Rolink, AG, Radaszkiewicz, T and Gleichmann, H (1984). Graft-versus-host reactions: clues to the etiopathology of a spectrum of immunological diseases. Immunol Today, 5, 324-32

33. Maurer, T, Thomann, P, Weinch, EG and Hess, R (1975). The optimization test in the guinea pig. Toxicology, 15, 163-71

34. Marzulli, FN and Maguire, HC Jr. (1982). Usefulness and

limitations of various guinea pig methods in detecting human
sensitizers. Fd Cosmet Toxicol, 16, 59-62
35. Miller, K, Maisey, J and Malkovsky, M (1984). Enhancement of
contact sensitization in mice fed a diet enriched in vitamin A
acetate. Int Arch Allergy Appl Immunol, 75, 120-5
36. Benson, MD and Aldo-Benson, M (1979). Effect of purified
protein SAA on immune responses in vitro: mechanisms of
suppression. J Immunol, 122, 2077-82
37. Feldman, G (1982). Synthesis and secretion of acute phase
proteins by the hepatocytes from rats with normal liver or
cirrhosis during the inflammatory reaction. Ann NY Acad Sci,
381, 446-7
38. Luster, MI, Dean, JH and Moore, JA (1982). Evaluation of
immune functions in toxicology. In Hayes, AW (ed). Methods
in Toxicology. pp.561-586. (New York: Raven Press)
39. van Furth, R (1976). An approach to the characterization of
mononuclear phagocytes involved in pathological processes.
Agents Actions, 6, 91-8
40. Nelson, DJ, Kiremidjian-Scheimacher, L and Stotsky, G
(1982). Effects of cadmium, lead and zinc on macrophage-
mediated cytoxicity toward tumor cells. Environ Res, 28, 154-
63
41. Miller, K and Brown, RC (1985). The immune system and asbestos associated disease. In Dean, JH, Munson, AE, Luster,
MI and Amos, HE (eds) Toxicology of the Immune System,
Target Organ Toxicity Series. pp.429-440 (New York: Raven
Press)
42. Fisher, GL, McNeill, KL and Democko, J (1983). Application
of bovine macrophage bioassays in the analysis of toxic agents
in complex environmental mixtures. In Waters, MD, Sandhu,
SF, Lewtas, J, Claxton, L, Charmoff, N and Nesnow, S
(eds). Short-term Bioassays in the Analysis of Complex Environmental Mixtures. Vol.III, pp.257-268. (New York:
Plenum)
43. Nagata, Y, Diamond, B and Bloom, BR (1983). The generation
of human monocyte/macrophage cell lines. Nature Lond, 306,
597-9
44. Feldman, M and Shreier, MH (1982). Monoclonal T cells and
their Products (New York: Academic Press)
45. Pfizenmaier, K, Scheurich, P, Daubener, W, Kronke, M, Rol-
linghoff, M and Wagner, H (1984). Quantitative representation
of all T cells committed to develop into cytoxic effector cells
and/or interleukin 2 activity-producing helper cells within
murine T lymphocyte subsets. Eur J Immunol, 14, 33-9
46. Henderson, LE, Hewetson, JF, Hopkins (III), RF, Sowder,
RC, Neubauer, RH and Rabin, H (1983). A rapid large scale
purification procedure for gibbon interleukin 2. J Immunol,
131, 810-15
47. Braun, J and Unanue, ER (1980). B lymphocyte biology
studied with anti-Ig antibodies. Immunol Rev, 52, 3-28
48. Ward, PA, Unanue, ER, Goralnick, SJ and Schreiner, GF
(1977). Chemotaxis of rat lymphocytes. J Immunol, 119, 416-21
49. Webster, D, Arlett, CF, Harcourt, SA, Teo, I and Henderson, L (1981). In Bridges, BA and Harnden, DG (eds)

Ataxia-Telangiectasia - A Cellular and Molecular Link between Cancer, Neuropathology and Immune Deficiency. pp.379-86. (London: John Wiley)

50.   Harris, G, Lawley, PD and Olsen, I (1981). Mode of action of methylating carcinogens in comparative studies of murine and human cells. Carcinogenesis, 2, 403-11

51.   Lumb, JR (1983). The value of theoretical models in immunological research. Immunol Today, 4, 209-10

14
Genetic Toxicology Testing

B. J. DEAN

INTRODUCTION

During the 1970s an intensive research effort was devoted to the development of techniques to investigate chemical-induced genetic damage in a variety of cells and organisms. The impetus for this research was provided, in the first place, by the realization that chemicals were capable of producing mutations in mammalian cells that may eventually increase the incidence of heritable disease in man and, secondly, the desire to find quick and inexpensive assays to detect chemicals with carcinogenic potential. Mutations are usually the result of an interaction of the chemicals with DNA, and it was generally accepted that the cellular changes associated with chemical-induced neoplasia were also responses to an interaction with DNA. It is now evident that, although the initial stages of neoplastic transformation probably require a change in DNA structure caused by a mutagenic carcinogen, other carcinogens do not react directly with DNA and exert their effects on other stages of the carcinogenic process, e.g. carcinogen enhancers[1]. Thus most of the current short-term assays for mutagenic and carcinogenic chemicals are based on interaction with DNA resulting in gene mutations, chromosomal aberrations, unscheduled DNA synthesis, etc. Such assays do not usually respond to non-genotoxic carcinogens including tumour promoters and other enhancers.

In excess of 100 test systems for investigating genotoxic chemicals have been described in the literature, ranging through the biological phyla from bacteriophage to mammals. Of these, fewer than 20 are in regular use and most of these are for specific investigations rather than routine testing of chemicals. The selection of the eight or so assays now in routine use has been based on (a) their utility and availability in testing laboratories, (b) the requirements of various regulatory agencies, and (c) their performance in a series of national and international validation studies.

It is almost universal practice to use short-term tests for genotoxic chemicals in batteries that detect more than one type of genetic change. Assays that utilize bacteria are the most widely used and most thoroughly validated, e.g. the Salmonella/microsomal assay introduced by Professor Bruce Ames[2]. In addition to a bacterial assay, an initial test battery may include tests for the detection of chromosome aberrations, gene mutations or unscheduled DNA synthesis in cultured mammalian cells, or genetic changes in yeast cultures or in the fruit fly, Drosophila melanogaster. These so-called screening tests are used basically to study the ability of a chemical to induce genetic damage. Following the detection of genotoxic activity it is usual to investigate the activity of the chemical in whole animal systems using assays for chromosome damage in somatic or germ cells, for DNA damage, e.g. unscheduled DNA synthesis in rodent hepatocytes, or for somatic mutations in mouse skin using the mouse spot test. The selection, application and interpretation of the currently accepted tests for genotoxic chemicals have been reviewed by a number of workers[3-5], and more detailed texts have been published[6-8].

Two recent international collaborative studies have had a significant impact on the use and selection of short-term tests. The first study[9], in which 42 established carcinogens or presumptive non-carcinogens were tested in some 30 different in vitro or in vivo assays in more than 50 laboratories, showed that the Salmonella/microsomal assay produced the best overall performance in discriminating between carcinogens and non-carcinogens. Even then, some carcinogens were not detected, or gave ambiguous results with the standard bacterial assay. The second study[10] was designed to identify assays that could detect these chemicals, and thus would complement the bacterial assay in a two-test battery. A battery consisting of a bacterial mutation test and an assay for chromosome aberrations in cultured cells is now widely accepted as the most useful for initial screening of chemicals for genotoxicity.

Current effort in the field of genotoxicity testing is concentrated on rationalizing the use of short-term tests and on the refinement of existing procedures. However, such are the recognized shortcomings of the existing assays for detecting carcinogens that considerable research is being devoted to developing more reliable, relevant and sensitive procedures. It is anticipated that the most significant developments will be in the isolation and characterization of new, metabolically competent cell lines to overcome the problems associated with the use of exogenous metabolic activation supplements in many assays. Secondly, there will be renewed efforts to introduce animal models and suitable techniques for investigating organic-specific genotoxicity in short-term studies in an attempt to reduce the need for long-term bioassays for the definitive identification of animal carcinogens. Techniques are also being introduced for monitoring industrial populations exposed to very low concentrations of genotoxic chemicals and for identifying susceptible individuals in exposed groups. Recombinant DNA technology will almost certainly influence the way in which carcinogens are studied during the next decade, and finally, computer technology may, at last, provide a reliable means of relating chemical structure to biological activity.

REFINEMENT OF EXISTING PROCEDURES

As discussed above, the Salmonella/microsomal assay and the in vitro mammalian cell cytogenic assay are the most widely used and better-validated short-term tests. There have been a number of attempts to modify the standard Ames technique either using a preincubation technique[11] or by replacing the conventional rat liver microsomal activation system with liver extracts from other species[12], but any overall improvement has been unremarkable. However, a critical appraisal of the in vitro chromosome assay resulted in recommendations that should improve its sensitivity, selectivity and reproducibility[13]. It was apparent, for some carcinogens, that the usual rat liver microsomal supplement was ineffective in the generation of clastogenic metabolites. Protocols providing experimental conditions that allowed optimum activity of the target cell's endogenous activating enzymes led to the detection of chromosome aberrations. In the short-term, therefore, the main emphasis in genetic toxicology testing will be in the critical evaluation of the protocols and the introduction of modifications and standardization that should improve their reliability and reproducibility between laboratories.

DEVELOPMENT OF MAMMALIAN CELL CULTURE SYSTEMS

With few exceptions the mammalian cell lines used to study gene mutations, chromosome damage and neoplastic transformation lack adequate mixed-function oxidase activity for the conversion of most genotoxic chemicals to reactive electrophiles. Cell types such as Chinese hamster ovary (CHO), Chinese hamster lung (V79), used for gene mutation and chromosome studies and mouse C3H 10T 1/2 and Balb/C 3T3 fibroblasts used in in vitro transformation assays, require supplementation with an exogenous source of metabolizing activity. This is usually introduced in the form of the S9 supernatant from a liver homogenate obtained from rats pre-treated with Arochlor[2]. Even this supplement does not provide for optimum activation of many carcinogens and, as discussed above, some chemicals can only be detected in mammalian cells when the protocol is modified to enhance the activity of endogenous bioactivation. There is therefore a need to isolate cell lines that retain a high level of native mixed-function oxidase and related enzyme activity, and to develop culture media and techniques that encourage the maintenance of metabolically competent cells for long periods of repeated subculture. Epithelial-type cells isolated from weaning rat liver retain substantial enzyme activity up to about 30 passages in culture[14,15] although maintenance of this activity requires great care with the subculture procedure. Danford[16] described a cell line derived from Chinese hamster liver that activated carcinogens such as acrylonitrile, ortho-toluidine, hexamethylphosphoramide and diethylstilbestrol to clastogenic metabolites. It is anticipated that metabolically competent cells of this type will receive considerable attention during the next few years, thus removing the need to supplement in vivo mammalian cell assays with liver microsomal preparations.

A variety of cell culture systems are used to investigate chemical-induced neoplastic transformation, and three of these are in fairly widespread use. Two of them, mouse C3H 10T 1/2[17] and Balb/C 3T3[18] fibroblasts suffer from the lack of adequate enzyme activity described above. Syrian hamster embryo (SHE) cells, however, are used as primary or secondary cultures and contain a high level of biotransformation activity. Thus they appear to be very suitable for characterizing carcinogenic and non-carcinogenic chemicals without the need for an exogenous enzyme supplement[19].

Most of the currently available short-term tests are designed to detect compounds that interact with DNA and only respond to genotoxic carcinogens, i.e. carcinogens that exert their activity through a non-genotoxic mechanism will not be detected in these assays. Increasing effort is being devoted to developing new procedures to investigate chemicals that modify pre-existing DNA lesions, e.g. tumour-enhancers and promoters. Experimental evidence indicates an association between tumour promotion and the induction of mitotic aneuploidy[20,21]. This is usually caused by an interaction of the chemical with elements of the mitotic spindle apparatus. A technique has been described[16] in which chemically induced mitotic aneuploidy can be readily detected in cultures of Chinese hamster liver cells.

Modified assays for neoplastic transformation are also being introduced in which cells are treated with a mutagenic chemical, usually a simple alkylating agent; at a concentration that does not induce transformed clones[22]. Subsequent treatment of these "initiated" cells with tumour promoters leads to detectable transformation, thus providing a promising assay for non-genotoxic tumour modifiers.

Significant progress is evident, therefore, in the development of metabolically competent cell lines and in the introduction of mammalian cell techniques for the detection of non-genotoxic carcinogens.

INVESTIGATION OF ORGAN-SPECIFIC GENOTOXICITY

Few chemical carcinogens appear to be fully multipotential in that they rarely induce neoplasms indiscriminately throughout the organism. On the contrary many agents, e.g. vinyl chloride, benzene, nitrosamines, are highly specific in their choice of target organ. In vitro assays simply describe a basic property of the test chemical, i.e. the chemical or its metabolite(s) is capable of interaction with DNA to produce mutations, chromosome aberrations, etc. The extrapolation of in vitro assays to whole animal carcinogenicity assumes that the chemical in question is capable of exerting its genotoxicity in vivo. If this assumption is accepted, then it is logical to predict that the same genetic changes are induced in the target organ for tumour formation. There is increasing interest in developing techniques in which experimental animals are given acute or sub-chronic doses of the test chemical and, after an appropriate period, possible target organs are isolated and established in primary culture. Cells from the target organs are then available for the study of a variety of genetic and other cellular changes.

The author[23] demonstrated the feasibility of this approach using Chinese hamsters. Animals were given single oral doses of the test chemical, and after a few hours the lung, liver, kidney, bladder and forestomach were prepared for primary culture. Using the HGPRT/8-azaguanine-resistance mutation system, a good correlation was observed between mutation induction in organs of Chinese hamsters and the organ distribution of neoplasms in rodents with 2-acetylaminofluorene, 3-methylcholanthrene, diethylnitrosamine and methylnitrosourea. With improved cell culture techniques it is now quite feasible to use this approach to study gene mutations, chromosome aberrations, sister chromatid exchange and unscheduled DNA synthesis in primary cultures from treated animals, and, eventually to detect neoplastic transformation. The development of transformation assays in primary cultures offers exciting possibilities. For example, one can induce the initial DNA lesion by treatment in vivo and then study the effects of various enhancers in cells cultured from the treated animal. Such a technique offers the possibility of investigating a test agent for both tumour-initiating and promoting activity in a specific target organ. To carry this concept a stage further, the application of recombinant DNA technology may allow the identification and characterization of specific cellular gene changes associated with transformation leading to the development of a very sophisticated short-term test for carcinogenic chemicals.

MONITORING HUMAN EXPOSURE TO GENOTOXIC CHEMICALS

The most common biological technique used to monitor the exposure of industrial populations to genotoxic chemicals is the analysis of peripheral blood lymphocytes for chromosomal changes. The method has been used in a variety of industries; increases in the frequency of chromosome aberrations have been reported in workers exposed to such chemicals as benzene[24], vinyl chloride[25] and ethylene oxide[26]. With recent improvements in industrial hygiene following legislation to limit exposure to many chemicals, current biological monitoring techniques lack the sensitivity required to detect exposure to low concentrations of these compounds.

A new tool for biological monitoring became available with the development of techniques to identify and measure specific adducts in informational and other biological macromolecules. Ehrenberg's group[27] correlated the occurrence of hydroxyethylated N-7-guanine in DNA and protein isolated from various organs after exposure of mice to ethylene oxide. The same workers also investigated the alkylation of haemoglobin as a monitor of exposure to certain agents[28,29]. Wright[30] has described refinements of this technique in studies that confirmed the value of haemoglobin-adduct analysis as a measure of adducts in DNA after exposure to ethylene oxide. A uniform level of hydroxyethylated N-7-guanine was observed from a wide range of tissues from ethylene oxide-treated rats. The only exception was testicular DNA which contained approximately half the amount of alkylation of other tissues. The uniformity of the response in various tissues in the rat suggests that there are unlikely to be significant variations in the correlation between ethylene oxide dose and tissue DNA dose of ethylene oxide in different mammals[30].

Earlier methods of detecting DNA adducts required radiolabelled test material. "Cold" methods, using gas chromatography and mass spectroscopy, have been developed[31], but are laborious, and the major advance in this field has been the introduction of immunochemical methods. The development of high-affinity antibodies to DNA adducts of alkylating agents[32-32], polycyclic aromatic hydrocarbons[35] and aromatic amines[34,36] have opened the way for the introduction of practical monitoring procedures for specific environmental chemicals in man. Providing experimental evidence is available for the correlation between haemoglobin dose, tissue DNA dose and exposure dose, i.e. as for ethylene oxide[30], then monitoring of peripheral blood haemoglobin is feasible. Alternatively, direct monitoring of DNA adducts in peripheral blood lymphocytes may be used[37]. Highly specific monoclonal antibodies can be used to detect DNA adducts at the single cell level using immunofluorescence microscopy, and this method has been applied successfully to various organs of rats treated with 2-acetylaminofluorene[38]. Poirier[39] has summarized a number of early successes with this technology and, using polyclonal and monoclonal antibodies to the major benzo(α)pyrene-DNA adducts, such adducts have been detected in DNA of lung tissues or peripheral blood leukocytes from lung cancer patients, and in leukocytes of roofers, foundry workers and cigarette smokers.

POPULATION HETEROGENEITY - VARIABILITY IN RESPONSE TO GENOTOXIC CHEMICALS

The immunochemical technology described above will also have important applications in the identification of individuals particularly susceptible to specific chemicals. Health and safety legislation governing exposure to environmental agents requires that exposure levels are defined so as to protect individuals who are highly susceptible to those agents. In practice, this usually means a 100- or 1000-fold safety margin between doses that induce toxicity in a laboratory animal model, and the permitted level in the environment, i.e. there are few methods currently available to identify susceptible individuals. Recent advances in the areas of pharmacogenetics, i.e. individual variation in the metabolism of particular drugs, and ecogenetics, i.e. individual variation in response to chemicals and other environmental agents, offer techniques that should eventually allow susceptible individuals to be identified, the degree of susceptibility to be measured, and should lead to a more precise definition of non-hazardous dose. Knowledge of the factors responsible for increased susceptibility may allow earlier recognition of individuals affected by chemical exposure and earlier efforts to control exposure to the offending chemical in the working environment. The prime importance of the cytochromes

P_{450} in the biotransformation of both foreign and endogenous chemicals has concentrated efforts to define the specific forms responsible for the detoxification and activation of various carcinogens and to characterize the inter-individual variation in the enzymes that result in increased susceptibility. A number of cytochromes P_{450} responsible for specific carcinogen reactions have been identified using monoclonal antibody techniques[40].

An example of the influence of genetic variability in cytochromes P_{450} is shown by the hypersensitive drug debrisoquine, which is readily metabolized to 4-hydroxydebrisoquine. About 10% of the population excrete very small quantities of this metabolite and Price-Evans et al[41] have shown that impaired debrisoquine metabolism is an autosomal recessive trait. P_{450} activity towards other substrates is usually normal, and it is presumed that incomplete hydroxylation of the drug is caused by an impaired P_{450} isozyme[42].

The factors that determine metabolic fate of a chemical and the availability of the ultimate toxic molecule to the molecular target are extremely complex. The compound specificity, inducibility and competitive inhibition of the cytochromes P_{450} alone suggest that the characterization of the metabolic routes responsible for the population variability in response to more than a few environmental agents and pharmaceuticals is a daunting task. Immunological technology will have a significant impact on the identification of individuals susceptible to certain chemicals without the need to characterize metabolic pathways. For compounds whose ultimate reactants are electrophiles, and whose cellular target is DNA or other macromolecules, the development of techniques to identify and quantify specific adducts offers a practical technique for identifying susceptible individuals. Such techniques are, at the moment, only useful for application to populations who are already exposed to a particular chemical, i.e. they identify the molecular consequence of exposure rather than the factors that determine susceptibility. After further development and evaluation monoclonal antibody techniques of this kind will almost certainly be the method of choice for monitoring industrial populations for exposure to low levels of genotoxic chemicals and for the detection of individuals unusually susceptible to these agents.

THE IMPACT OF RECOMBINANT DNA TECHNOLOGY ON GENETIC TOXICOLOGY

The past few years have witnessed tremendous advances in the use of recombinant DNA technology in the study of the specific genes associated with neoplasia and in the characterization of mutations at the gene level. As a result these techniques will play a vital role in the evolution of short-term testing for mutagens and carcinogens. An excellent review of the application of DNA technology to the study of genes and gene alterations has been prepared by the International Commission for Protection against Environmental Mutagens and Carcinogens[43].

Evidence that specific genes were responsible for neoplastic transformation of mammalian cells was provided by the observation that acute transforming RNA viruses, i.e. retroviruses, contain genes that, when inserted into the mammalian cell genome, resulted in neoplastic transformation. These specific transforming genes are called oncogenes. The viral oncogenes are almost identical to certain normal cellular genes and can be inserted into cellular DNA with relative ease using transfection techniques. They can be characterized by restriction enzyme analysis[43]. A number of different cellular genes have been implicated in the development of neoplasms[44]. They are referred to as cellular transforming genes or co-oncogenes (to differentiate them from the v-oncogenes of retroviruses) and have been identified by transfection assays or by their similarity to the transforming genes of retroviruses. Many of the earlier studies on cellular transforming genes used the mouse fibroblast cell line, NIH/3T3, which can be phenotypically transformed by transfection with DNA fragments from tumour cells[45].

Using DNA fragments isolated from cell lines derived from human bladder carcinomas, it has been shown by transfection studies, in NIH/3T3 cells, that the ras oncogene responsible for neoplastic transformation differs only by a single base-pair substitution from the oncogenes of normal bladder cells[46-48]. However, NIH/3T3 is an established, i.e. immortalized, cell line, generally regarded as preneoplastic. Transformation by a single mutated ras oncogene may therefore only reflect the final stage of transformation. It appears that an essential step in the transformation process is the immortalization of cells, and the activation of at least two oncogenes are required for progression to overt transformation. This is supported by studies demonstrating that transformation of primary rodent fibroblast cultures required activation of both the ras and myc oncogenes, and that activation of ras was a result of a base-pair substitution and myc activation was associated with a specific DNA rearrangement[49]. Thus a picture is beginning to emerge of an association between the activation of specific cellular oncogenes (by mutation, DNA rearrangement or, possibly, mitotic aneuploidy) and a multistage transformation process. The present status of oncogene research is reviewed by Cooper and Lane[44].

Oncogene activation leads either to a qualitative change resulting in an abnormal gene product or to a quantitative increase in the normal gene product. In principle quantitative immunochemical techniques can recognize the products of either of these changes. Providing the cellular transforming genes in a model cell culture system are fully characterized and monoclonal antibodies can be produced to measure both normal and abnormal oncogene products, then a practicable assay for detecting changes in activity of each oncogene would be available. Such an assay would not require the demonstration of a neoplastic phenotype, and offers the exciting possibility of detecting the chemical-induced activation of oncogenes concerned with initiating events and those involved with progressive stages to overt neoplasia. The cell lines currently used in transformation assays, such as mouse fibroblast C3H 10T 1/2 and BalbC 3T3, are generally accepted as partly transformed or preneoplastic and to provide an acceptable assay for the oncogenes mediating each stage of transformation, development of procedures based on primary cell types will be necessary.

The influence of recombinant DNA technology on mutagenicity testing is more difficult to foresee. The gene changes associated with mutational events can now be characterized and their location in the genome identified. This may lead to the comparison of gene changes in germ cells with those in the cellular targets of mutagenicity assays using, for example, bone marrow cells, which may confirm or invalidate the value of somatic cell data for predicting germ cell mutations[43]. It may also be instructive to integrate specific mammalian genes into a microbial genome in order to study the effects of chemicals on these genes in very simple experimental systems. There is also the interesting possibility of dissecting and characterizing the genes that control the very complex mammalian DNA repair systems and using this information to construct experimental systems in which human DNA syndromes could be studied or which could be used to investigate the influence of DNA repair on the fate of pre-mutational lesions in DNA[43].

STRUCTURE-ACTIVITY CONSIDERATIONS: ARTIFICIAL INTELLIGENCE

Literature searched before 1985 contained references to at least 10,000 chemicals that had been tested in short-term genotoxity assays[50]. Not surprisingly the quality of these data is variable, and one objective of the US Environmental Protection Agency Gene-Tox Program was to assess the data and select those that met predetermined criteria of quality[50], i.e. about 40% of the published data[50]. The acceptable data from compounds tested in a number of the assays were computer-coded and a preliminary analysis showed that, although most chemical classes were represented, there were only a few chemicals in each class and many chemicals had been tested in only a few assays. Evaluation of the assays in terms of the prediction of carcinogenic potential was limited by the small number of chemicals on which animal cancer data were available. It seemed, therefore, that the tremendous investment in short-term tests had yielded little of direct value to help the selection of assays that would reliably detect animal carcinogens.

After assessing these data, Rosenkranz and his colleagues[50] devised a series of computer programs aimed at relating chemical structures to biological activity. The first of these, referred to as Computer-Automated Structure Evaluation (CASE), uses an artificial intelligence method that is capable of scanning molecular structures and suggesting possible active, e.g. electrophilic, sites. The CASE program generates the correct bonding between given atoms introduced into the structure, and an additional program is able to generate three-dimensional geometry for each molecule. The system is capable of identifying each potentially active or inactive sub-unit in a molecule using the data base of biological activity selected by the Gene-Tox Program. It can therefore analyse an unknown molecule and project its expected genotoxic activity. For example, when nitroarenes were analysed, four subunits were identified, two of which are associated with mutagenic activity and two that are deactivating. Nitroarenes that contain one of the "active" subunits are mutagenic, while those that lack these sub-units or contain a deactivating sub-unit are inactive in short-term tests[50].

One of the ultimate goals of this project is to characterize a battery of short-term tests most suitable for the detection of animal carcinogens. The structure-activity data generated from the program should allow the selection of assays based on their ability to detect active sub-units in molecules of diverse structure. Its main value, however, may be in reducing the number of chemicals that need to be tested in either short-term assays and long-term cancer bioassays. Once it is established that the data base of biological activity is adequate, chemicals that are reliably predicted as genotoxic by the CASE program should not require testing, and the available genetic toxicology resources can then be devoted to classes for which biological data are inadequate.

Needless to say there are major shortcomings in this imaginative approach, and they are associated with the failings of the currently available short-term tests and the variable quality of published carcinogenity data. As discussed earlier in this chapter, most of the present in vitro assays depend on an exogenous source of metabolism that is not appropriate to all chemical classes and, in general, they detect activity associated with DNA dama, i.e. they fail to identify tumour promoters and other enhancers. This is an added incentive to develop short-term procedures that will respond to "non-genotoxic" carcinogens using techniques that eliminate the need for exogenous activation systems.

DISCUSSION: THE FUTURE

For almost a decade bacterial mutation assays have formed the backbone of short-term testing for mutagens and carcinogens. For reasons discussed above, bacterial and related assays are not sufficiently reliable for the prediction of animal carcinogenic activity. It is inevitable that bacterial assays will continue in use for some time yet, but equally inevitable that some of the new approaches to detecting carcinogens will prove sufficiently reliable and cost-effective to supercede most of the current generation of tests after the end of this decade.

It is anticipated that the most significant improvements in current technology will lead to the establishment of mammalian, preferably human, cell lines cultured in an environment that maintains the metabolic, structural and genomic features of the primary cells in continuous culture over long periods. Simple and fully characterized assays for gene mutation at a range of loci will remove the need for bacterial models so that the next generation of screening assays for genotoxicity will comprise systems that detect gene mutation and structural and numerical chromosome aberrations in mammalian cells. Assays for morphological evidence of neoplastic transformation in metabolically competent cell cultures will also become widely available. In vivo assays should keep pace with developments in cell culture procedures. Techniques to study the full spectrum of genetic changes, including DNA adducts, in cultures isolated from the major organs of animals treated with test materials are now quite feasible, and should permit a comprehensive investigation of organ-specific genotoxicity with a minimal outlay in animal resources and time.

The useful life of these second-generation assays will depend to a large extent on the pace of the application of the "new" technologies to genetic toxicology. As discussed earlier in this chapter, recombinant DNA techniques are even now at a stage where the design of neoplastic transformation assays based on the detection and measurement of cellular transforming gene products is possible. The potential rewards of recombinant DNA technology in commercially viable areas are very great, and little of the available expertise and few of the resources may be devoted to the development of specific techniques for screening chemicals. Equally rewarding, however, is the search for a definitive mechanism of cancer induction and progression, and appropriate short-term assays may be a spin-off from this research.

A combination of recombinant DNA methods and DNA adduct analysis may eventually answer one of the most perplexing and important questions in genetic toxicology - the establishment of genotoxic thresholds. These are usually estimated by extending dose-response curves generated from germ cell mutation studies or cancer studies in laboratory animals and the presence or absence of threshold doses of mutagens or carcinogens has been a constant source of argument. Analysis of DNA sequences in germ cells from treated animals should provide definitive evidence of mutagenic activity and the measurement of DNA adducts at a range of doses of the test material should provide the ultimate dose-response curve. Such data could provide indisputable evidence for the presence or absence of a threshold, and will be of fundamental importance to genotoxic risk assessment.

DNA adduct analysis has another application of equal value in aiding the extrapolation of animal bioassay data to human risk assessment[30]. With the development of techniques for maintaining the metabolic integrity of in vitro tissue preparations from experimental animals, the tissue distribution of DNA adducts to specific genotoxic agents can be established both in vivo and in the in vitro model. Characterization of the adduct profile in a range of experimental species will permit the development of in vitro models from human tissues, e.g. skin explants, blood leukocytes and autopsy samples of other organs, in which the pattern of DNA adducts may be used to predict the adduct distribution in human tissues in vivo. In addition to providing a sound basis for estimating the human risk associated with exposure to a given dose of an animal carcinogen, such techniques may be able to indicate the most susceptible target organ(s) and assist in the clinical surveillance of exposed populations.

The application of artificial intelligence to genetic toxicology presents the most intriguing and exciting possibility of all[50]. At the present rate of testing, and given the anticipated technological developments, it appears very likely that by the end of the century there will be sufficient biological data from enough members of all chemical classes to enable the genotoxic activity of novel molecules to be determined simply by entering the molecular structure into a central data bank. These techniques are not confined to genetic toxicology and one can envisage the 21st-century toxicologist obtaining a complete toxicology profile without leaving his computer terminal.

REFERENCES

1. Clayson, DB (1981). Carcinogens and carcinogen enhancers. ICPEMC Working Paper No.2/3. Mutation Res., 86, 217-29
2. Ames, BN, McCann, J and Yamasaki, E (1975). Methods for detecting carcinogens and mutagens with the Salmonella/mammalian microsome mutagenicity test. Mutation Res, 31, 347-64
3. Butterworth, B and Goldberg, L (eds)(1979). Strategies for Short-term Tests for Mutagens and Carcinogens. (West Palm Beach, Florida: CRC Press)
4. Department of Health and Social Security: Committee on Mutagenicity of Chemicals in Food, Consumer Products and the Environment (1981). Guidelines for the Testing of Chemicals for Mutagenicity. (London: HMSO)
5. Dean, BJ and Hodges, P (1982). Short-term tests for genotoxicity. In Balls, M, Riddell, RJ and Worden, AN (eds) Animals and Alternatives in Toxicity Testing. pp.381-409. (London: Academic Press)
6. Brustick, D (1980). Principles of Genetic Toxicology. (New York/London: Plenum Press)
7. United Kingdom Environmental Mutagen Society (1983). Report of the UKEMS Sub-Committee on Guidelines for Mutagenicity Testing, Part 1. Dean, BJ (ed). (University of Swansea: UKEMS)
8. United Kingdom Environmental Mutagen Society (1084). Report of the UKEMS Sub-Committee on Guidelines for Mutagenicity Testing, Part 2. Dean, BJ (ed). (University of Swansea: UKEMS)
9. De Serres, FJ and Ashby, J (eds)(1982). Evaluation of Short-term Tests for Carcinogens. Progress in Mutation Research, Vol.1. (Amsterdam: Elsevier)
10. Ashby, J, de Serres, FJ, Draper, M, Ishidate, M (Jnr), Margolin, B, Matter, B and Shelby, MD (eds)(1985). Evaluation of Short-term Tests for Carcinogens: Report of the International Program on Chemical Safety Collaborative Study on In Vitro Assays. (Amsterdam: Elsevier)
11. Brooks, TM and Dean, BJ (1982). Mutagenic activity of 42 coded compounds in the Salmonella/microsome assay with preincubation. In de Serres, FJ and Ashby, J (eds) Evaluation of Short-term Tests for Carcinogens. Progress in Mutation Research, Vol. 1. pp.261-70. (Amsterdam: Elsevier)
12. Venitt, S and Forster, R (1985). Bacterial mutagenicity assays: co-ordinators' report. In Arlett, CF and Parry, JM (eds) Comparative Genetic Toxicology: The Second UKEMS Collaborative Study. (London: Macmillan)
13. Dean, BJ (1985). Summary report on the performace of cytogenetic assays in cultured mammalian cells. In Ashby, J,

de Serres, FJ, Draper, M, Ishidate, M (Jnr), Margolin, BH, Matter, BE and Shelby, MD (eds) Evaluation of Short-term Tests for Carcinogens: Report of the International Program on Chemical Safety Collaborative Study on In Vitro Assays. pp.69-83. (Amsterdam: Elsevier)

14. Dean, BJ and Hodson-Walker, G (1979). An in vitro chromosome assay using cultured rat liver cells. Mutation Res, 64, 329-37

15. Tong, C and Williams, GM (1978). Induction of purine analog-resistant mutants in adult rat liver epithelial lines by metabolic activation-dependant and -independant carcinogens. Mutation Res, 58, 339-52

16. Danford, ND (1985). Tests for chromosomal aberrations and aneuploidy in the Chinese hamster fibroblast line CH1-L. In Ashby, J, de Serres, FJ, Draper, M, Ishidate, M (Jnr), Margolin, BH, Matter, BE and Shelby, MD (eds). Evaluation of Short-term Tests for Carcinogens: Report of the International Program on Chemical Safety Collaborative Study on In Vitro Assays. pp.397-411. (Amsterdam: Elsevier)

17. Marquardt, H, Juroki, T, Huberman, E, Selkirk, JK, Heidelberger, C, Grover, PL and Sims, P (1972). Malignant transformation of cells derived from mouse prostate by epoxides and other derivatives of polycyclic hydrocarbons. Cancer Res, 32, 716-20

18. DiPaolo, JA, Takano, K and Popescu, NC (1972). Quantitation of chemically induced neoplastic transformation of BALB/3T3 cloned cell lines. Cancer Res, 32, 2686-95

19. Pienta, RJ, Poiley, JA and Lebhertz, WB (1977). Morphological transformation of early passage golden Syrian hamster embryo cells derived from cryo-preserved primary cultures as a reliable in vitro assay for identifying diverse carcinogens. Int J Cancer, 19, 642-55

20. Parry, JM, Parry, EM and Barrett, JC (1981). Tumour promoters induce mitotic aneuploidy in yeast. Nature, 294, 263-65

21. Tsusui, T, Maizumi, H, McLachlan, JA and Barrett, JC (1983). Aneuploidy-induction and cell transformation by diethylstilbestrol: a possible chromosome mechanism in carcinogens. Cancer Res, 43, 3816-21

22. Meyer, AL (1983). In vitro transformation assays for chemical carcinogens. Mutation Res, 115, 323-38

23. Dean, BJ and Hodson-Walker, G (1979). Organ-specific mutations in Chinese hamsters induced by chemical carcinogens. Mutation Res, 64, 407-13

24. Dean, BJ (1985). Recent findings on the genetic toxicology of benzene, toluene, xylenes and phenols. Mutation Res (in press)

25. Purchase, IFH, Richardson, CR, Anderson, D, Paddle, GM and Adams, WGF (1978). Chromosomal analysis in vinyl chloride-exposed workers. Mutation Res, 57, 325-34

26. Laurent, C, Frederic, J and Marachal, F (1983). Increased sister chromatid exchange frequency in workers exposed to ethylene oxide. Ann Genet, 26, 138-42

27. Ehrenberg, L, Hiesche, KD, Osterman-Golkar, S and Wen-

nburg, I (1974). Evaluation of genetic risk of alkylating agents: tissue doses in the mouse from air contaminated with ethylene oxide. Mutation Res, 24, 83-103

28. Osterman-Golkar, S, Ehrenberg, L, Segerback, D and Hallstrom, I (1976). Evaluation of genetic risks of alkylating agents. II. Haemoglobin as a dose monitor. Mutation Res, 34, 1-10

29. Segerback, D, Calleman, CJ, Ehrenberg, L, Lofroth, G and Osterman-Golkar, S (1978). Evaluation of genetic risks of alkylating agents. IV. Quantitative determination of alkylated amino acids in haemoglobin as a measure of the dose after treatment of mice with methyl methane-sulphonate. Mutation Res, 49, 71-82

30. Wright, AS (1983). Molecular dosimetry techniques in human risk assessment: an industrial perspective. In Hayes, AW, Schnell, RC and Miya, TS (eds) Developments in the Science and Practice of Toxicology. pp.311-18. (Amsterdam: Elsevier)

31. Farmer, PB, Bailey, E, Lamb, JH and Connors, TA (1980). Approach to the quantitation of alkylated amino acids in haemoglobin by gas chromatography mass spectrometry. Biomed Mass Spectrom, 7, 41-7

32. Briscoe, WT, Spizizen, J and Tan, EM (1978). Immunological detection of O^6-methylguanine in alykylated DNA. Biochemistry, 17, 1896-1901

33. Rajewsky, MF, Muller, R, Adamkiewicz, J and Drosdziok, W (1980). Immunological detection and quantification of DNA components structurally modified by alkylating carcinogens (ethylnitrosourea). In Pullman, B, Ts'o, POP and Gelboin, H (eds) Carcinogenesis: Fundamental Mechanisms and Environmental Effects. pp.207-16. (Dordrecht: Reidel)

34. Van der Laken, CJ, Hagenaars, AM, Hermsen, G, Kriek, E, Kuipers, AJ, Nagel, J, Scherer, E and Welling, M (1982). Measurement of O^6-ethyldeoxyguanosine and N-(deoxy-guanosin-8-yl)-N-acetyl-2-amino-fluorene in DNA by high-sensitive enzyme immunoassays. Carcinogenesis, 5, 569-72

35. Poirier, MC, Santella, R, Weinstein, IB, Gruberger, D and Yuspa, SH (1980). Quantitation of benzo-α-pyrene-deoxy-guanosine adducts by radio-immunoassay. Cancer Res, 40, 412-16

36. Poirier, MC, Yuspa, SH, Weinstein, IB and Blobstein, S (1977). Detection of carcinogen-DNA adducts by radioim-munoassay. Nature Lond, 270, 186-8

37. Bean, RA, Schoen, MA, Zaalberg, OE and Lohman, PM (1982). The detection of DNA damage by immunological tech-niques. In Sorsa, MH and Vainio, H (eds) Mutagens in Our Environment. pp.111-24. (New York: Alan R. Liss)

38. Lohman, PHM (1985). Immunochemical detection of DNA ad-ducts in mammalian cells at the single cell level: a sensitive tool for biomonitoring purposes. Abstracts of the Fourteenth Annual Meeting of the European Environmental Mutagen Society. Mutation Res (in press)

39. Poirier, MC (1984). The use of carcinogen-DNA adduct an-tisera for quantitation and localisation of genomic damage in animal models and the human population. Environ Mutagen,

6, 879-87

40. Gelboin, HV, Fujino, T, Song, B-J, Park, SS, Cheng, K-C, West, D, Robinson, R, Miller, H and Friedman, FK (1984). Monoclonal antibody-directed phenotyping of cytochromes P-450 by enzyme inhibition, immunopurification and radioimmunoassays. In Omenn, GS and Gelboin, HV (eds) Genetic Variability in Responses to Chemical Exposure, Banbury Report 16. pp.65-84. (Cold Spring Harbor Laboratory)

41. Price-Evans, DA, Mahgoub, A, Sloan, TP, Idle, JR and Smith RL (1980). A family and population study of the genetic polymorphism of debrisoquine oxidation in a white British population. J Med Genet, 17, 102-10

42. Distlerath, LM, Larrey, D and Guengerich, FP (1984). Genetic polymorphism of debrisoquine 4-hydroxylation: identification of the defect at the level of a specific cytochrome P-450 in a rat model. In Omenn, GS and Gelboin, HV (eds) Genetic Variability in Responses to Chemical Exposure: Banbury Report 16. pp.85-96. (Cold Spring Harbor Laboratory)

43. Mekler, Ph, Delehanty, JT, Lohman, PHM, Brouwer, J, Putte, PvD, Pearson, P, Pouwels, PH and Ramel, C (1985). The use of recombinant DNA technology to study gene alteration; ICPEMC Publication No.11. Mutation Res (in press)

44. Cooper, GF and Lane, M-A (1984). Cellular transforming genes and oncogenesis. Biochim Biophys Acta, 738, 9-20

45. Shih, C, Shilo, BZ, Goldfarb, MP, Dannenberg, A and Weinberg, RA (1979). Passage of phenotypes of chemically transformed cells via transfection of DNA and chromatin. Proc Natl Acad Sci USA, 76, 5714-18

46. Reddy, EP, Reynolds, RK, Santos, E and Barbacid, M (1982). A point mutation is responsible for the acquisition of transforming properties by the T24 human bladder carcinoma oncogene. Nature, Lond, 300, 149-52

47. Tabin, CJ, Bradley, SM, Bargmann, CI, Weinberg, RA, Papageorge, AG, Scolnick, EM, Dhar, R, Lowy, DR and Chang EH (1982). Mechanism of activation of a human oncogene. Nature, Lond, 300, 143-9

48. Taporowsky, E, Suard, Y, Fasano, O, Shimizu, K, Goldfarb, M and Wigler, M (1982). Activation of the T24 bladder carcinoma transforming gene is linked to a single amino acid change. Nature, Lond, 300, 762-5

49. Land, H, Parada, LF and Weinberg, RA (1983). Tumorigenic conversion of primary embryo fibroblasts requires at least two cooperating oncogenes. Nature, Lond, 304, 596-602

50. Rosenkranz, HS, Klopman, G, Chankong, V, Pet-Edwards, J and Haimes, YY (1984). Prediction of environmental carcinogens: a strategy for the mid-1980s. Environ Mutagen, 6, 231-58

51. Waters, MD and Auletta, A (1981). The GENE-TOX Program: genetic activity evaluation. J Chem Inf Comput Sci, 21, 35-8

15

The Role of Dynamic Mathematical Models

E. R. CARSON

INTRODUCTION

In recent years there has been a significant increase in the use of dynamic mathematical models across the whole spectrum of life sciences and medicine. Initially the emphasis was on the the role of such models as research tools, whereas to an ever greater extent they can now serve as aids to the clinician in a wide range of situations relating to diagnosis and patient management. Of great potential is the use of dynamic mathematical models in predicting the response of the patient to therapy. In this brief chapter, trends in the predictive use of models will be discussed, particularly in relation to matters of safety evaluation.

DYNAMIC MODELLING METHODOLOGY

Making predictions of drug levels in the individual patient requires a clear quantitative understanding of the underlying metabolic dynamics as well as the relevant pharmacokinetics and pharmacodynamics. Fortunately, the methodology necessary for the development of dynamic mathematical models in the life sciences and medicine is now well defined[1].

The basis of the modelling approach is that many of the phenomena occurring in living organisms are fundamental physical and chemical processes which individually are more or less well known, and whose dynamic behaviour can be adequately described by appropriate mathematical equations. Where physiological processes are less well understood, mathematical equations can still in many cases be written; however in such cases they are formed empirically to describe dynamic data which are obtained experimentally. All these equations are then assembled together and programmed into a digital computer which then solves them, thereby producing a simulation of the behaviour of the real physiological system. Computer-based models can be used in this way to test hypotheses and gain further insight into the operation of complex dynamic biological processes.

The type of mathematical representation to be adopted for a particular model is critically dependent upon the purpose for which the model is intended. Examples of model purpose relevant to the analysis of drug effects include those given by Carson in 1983[2,3].

1. **Dose-response models.** Appropriate mathematical models can fulfil an important predictive role in relation to drug administration. Provided that they have been adequately validated, such models can be used to predict the response of the organism to varying doses of a particular drug, or conversely can be used to determine the dose pattern required to bring about a particular metabolic effect. This predictive use of modelling is discussed further below.

2. **Estimation of physiological parameters which cannot be measured directly.** Models can be used to make estimates of quantities such as fractional transfer rates, thereby enabling measures to be obtained for hepatic uptake of drugs and metabolites. Model-based parameter estimation can thus reduce the need for invasive animal experiments.

3. **Enhancing experimental design.** Models can be used in order to improve experimental design; for instance where the dynamic response of a physiological system is being defined following the administration of a radioisotopic tracer. Since experimental data in such cases are often obtained by counting radioactivity in blood samples withdrawn over a period of time, there is a limit imposed on the information that can be extracted as a result of limitations on sample size and frequency. Using appropriate models, sampling patterns can be optimized so as to obtain the maximum of information about the system from the minimum of blood samples.

PREDICTIVE MODELLING

Models which are soundly based upon the underlying physiological processes, rather than being simple statistical representations, can result in the prediction of clinical trends, and hence can be used to predict the effect of potentially therapeutic agents including consideration of their effectiveness and toxicity.

Mathematical models can be developed in this way at a number of levels: from the dynamics of subcellular effects to global models which consider the intact organism. Models which are associated with clinical measurement, however, are usually formulated at either the organ or global (intact organism) level. In a theoretical context this corresponds to a high degree of aggregation of the molecular, cellular and organ processes occurring within the organism.

An example of a model devised for clinical application and formulation in a manner which includes substantial unit process information in one of the human cardiovascular system intended for use in predicting the magnitude and pattern of the short-term effects of rapid acting drug therapy[4]. The model has three main sections: a model of the circulatory fluid mechanics, a neural control model and a pharmacokinetic model. Overall the model is soundly based on the underlying physiology, although within its three sections different degrees of aggregation, abstraction and idealization are apparent in the model formulation process. The circulatory fluid mechanics section is described mathematically in terms of the underlying physical laws. The neural control section, however, is less well understood, and thus whilst physiological relationships are preserved, a substantial degree of empiricism enters into the formulation. The pharmacodynamics section is partly physical and partly empirical. The basic approaches to pharmacokinetics and pharmacodynamic modelling are well established and have been widely summarized (see, for example, Whiting and Kelman[5]). This model was capable of predicting the overall effects on the cardiovascular system of drugs designed to regulate blood pressure during the 2-3 minute period following its administration.

A second example relates to the clinical modelling of fluid/electrolyte balance in order to predict the effects of therapy[6]. The physiologically based model provides representations of plasma, interstitial and intracellular fluids as appropriate in relation to water, protein, sodium, potassium, chloride, phosphate, organic acid, urea and carbon dioxide, together with the control effects of the hormones, ADH and aldosterone. As such it can first be used to obtain a greater understanding of the dynamics and control of the underlying physicochemical processes and to highlight areas of weak knowledge where additional data must be acquired before the models can be deemed to be of adequate validity for clinical purposes. The models can then be extended to encompass the abnormalities and malfunctions of fluid and electrolyte balance such as are associated with acutely ill patients receiving intensive therapy. The objectives include the use of model parameters estimated for the individual patient as a diagnostic index for that patient, and the use of the model as a predictor of the outcome of therapy, and hence a decision aid in patient management.

These two examples serve to illustrate the predictive role of physiologically based models. By tuning the parameters of such models to the individual subject or patient they can be used to predict the effects of drugs whose dynamics are also incorporated in the model. Thus the effect of variation of drug regime (dose, duration, frequency, etc.) on the individual over a period of time can be assessed. In this way dynamic mathematical models will increasingly find application in predictive safety evaluation.

THE ROLE OF ARTIFICIAL INTELLIGENCE

In the field of artificial intelligence there are now computer programs which simulate human knowledge and reasoning in specific disciplines up to an expert level. Such programs, which are often referred to as "expert systems", have profound implications for many areas of clinical medicine and are almost certain to impact upon predictive safety evaluation.

An expert system normally consists of a knowledge base and an interpreter or inference engine. The interpreter uses the knowledge base to make inferences from the information supplied by the user, often prompting for it in a consultative fashion.

The nature of expert systems makes obvious their application in a range of medical consultation situations. They have been developed to handle the more complex diagnostic and treatment cognitive tasks encountered by medical specialists and primary-care physicians. The fact that their knowledge base can encapsulate quantitative tests, logical inferences, rules-of-thumb, etc., means that they clearly have potential as aids to predictive safety evaluation.

Although their potential is great, it has to date been nothing like fully realized. This will change since researchers in artificial intelligence now have a much better understanding of the various knowledge representation schemes and methods of inference. Developments taking place in relation to both computer hardware and software will greatly facilitate the setting-up of expert systems to the extent that in the next decade they will be widely used in a range of areas relating to pharmacodynamics, pharmacotoxicity and safety evaluation.

DECISION SUPPORT SYSTEMS FOR PREDICTIVE SAFETY EVALUATION

It is highly desirable and most likely that during the next decade decision support systems for predictive safety evaluation will draw upon expert or knowledge-based systems from artificial intelligence and dynamic mathematical models of the underlying physicochemical processes of both patients and drugs or other therapeutic substances. As yet there has been only the beginnings of consideration of the possibility of incorporating all these elements into a single control model; all the dynamic, temporal and cognitive elements in a single decision support system[7]. Such knowledge-based systems with an empirical rule base in which simulation of knowledge and reasoning in terms of flow charts, production rules and verbal models incorporating networks of dose-effect relations, normally referred to as expert systems, have important implications for predictive safety evaluation. Such expert systems are symbolic models of human cognition with the ability to cope with uncertainty in knowledge and reasoning; modularity allowing ready correction and expansion; a human-like "friendly" interface to the user; and the ability to explain their own reasoning procedure. The quantitative predictive dynamic component will be derived from mathematical models.

Thus the new type of knowledge-based system on a decision aid will mesh an expert system as traditionally viewed with dynamic mathematical models. Properly designed and validated dynamic models will have an important role in determining what variables to measure, when to measure, and how to combine and transform data in order to yield information for safety evaluation.

REFERENCES

1. Carson, ER, Cobelli, C and Finkelstein, L (1983). Mathematical Modeling of Metabolic and Endocrine Systems. Model Formulation, Identification and Validation. (New York: Wiley)
2. Carson, ER (1983). The role of mathematical models in biomedical research. In Turner, P (ed.) Animals in Scientific Research: and Effective Substitute for Man? pp. 161-77
3. Carson, ER (1983). Mathematical models in pharmacotoxicity. In Balls, M, Riddell, R and Worden, AN (eds) Animals and Alternatives in Toxicity Testing. pp. 154-60. (London: Academic Press)
4. Leaning, MS, Pullen, HE, Carson, ER and Finkelstein, L (1983). Modelling a complex biological system: the human cardiovascular system. I. Methodology and model description. Trans Inst Meas Conr, 5, 71-86
5. Whiting, B and Kelman, AW (1985). Clinical decision making using pharmacokinetic and pharmacodynamic data. In Carson, ER and Cramp, DG (eds) Computers and Control in Clinical Medicine. pp. 59-93. (New York: Plenum)
6. Leaning, MS, Flood, RL, Cramp, DG and Carson, ER (1985). A system of models for fluid-electrolyte dynamics. IEEE Trans Biomed Eng, BME-32 (In press)
7. Cramp, DG and Carson, ER (1985). The patient/clinician relationship, computing and the wider health care system. In Carson, ER and Cramp, DG (eds) Computers and Control in Clinical Medicine. pp. 245-55. (New York: Plenum)

Index

INDEX

219